Take Your TASTEBUDS On A JOURNEY

A Neurodiverse-Friendly Cookbook

Spenser Duncan

WRITE AWAY

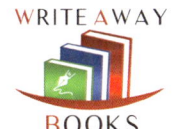

BOOKS

For information regarding discounts for bulk purchases or promotional applications of this book,
contact rob@writeawaybooks.com.

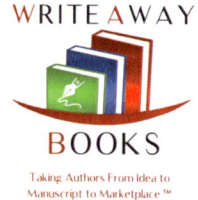

WRITE AWAY

BOOKS

Taking Authors From Idea to
Manuscript to Marketplace ™

Published by Write Away Books
PO Box 1681, Carlsbad, CA 92018
www.writeawaybooks.com

Book design by Beth Hutchins Design
Lakeside, CA

ISBN 979-8-9896431-7-2

First Edition

DEDICATION

I dedicate this cookbook to individuals with special needs who aspire to independence. A significant aspect of being independent is the ability to prepare your meals. This cookbook helps you reach your goals.

Thank you to all the family, teachers, and friends who helped me write this book. A special thank you to my dad, who taught me to cook; to my girlfriend, Connie, for letting me cook for her; to Mary for helping me write the recipes; to Master Sal Covento, of the United States Karate Academy in San Diego, for inspiring me to write this book; and to Brenda Goldbaum, who got me started and helped keep me organized as I began this project. I would also like to thank Rob, Beth, and Susan at Write Away Books, as well as Martin at the San Diego Regional Center, for making this all possible.

I never could have done this without all of you helping me.

~Spenser

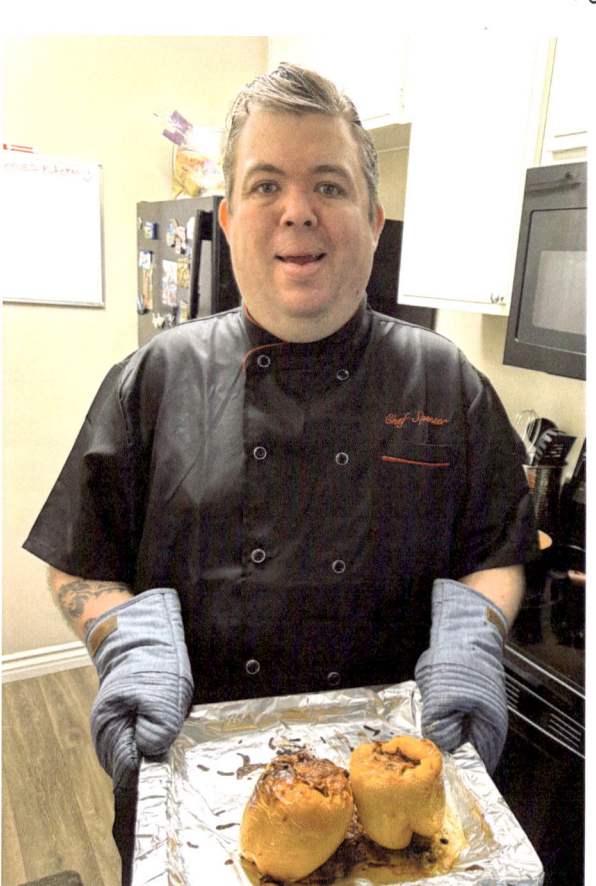

MY STORY

My name is Spenser Duncan, and I am 37 years old. I live in San Diego with my girlfriend, and I cook all of my meals. Cooking is a huge part of my life. For me, cooking is about more than just food–it's about independence.

When I was seven years old, I was diagnosed with a severe reading and writing disability. I graduated from high school, but getting through school was challenging. Throughout my life, cooking has been a constant source of joy. My dad taught me how to cook, and while he wasn't a fancy chef, he taught me all the basics and I have so many fond memories of us together in the kitchen whipping up pastas and different chicken dishes.

Ratatouille is one of my favorite movies because I'm just like the main character in the movie. I don't have one favorite spice or ingredient, I just like to do what feels good, and experiment to find the best flavors. My favorite dish to make is the San Marino pasta dish featured in this book; in fact, Marino is my middle name!

Cooking is important to me for so many reasons. I have lived on my own for 20 years, and being able to cook for myself is a huge milestone for someone like me to live independently. It's also a great way to save money. Cooking is also how I get to experience the world. I may not have the money to travel, but my taste buds sure do! When I make a dish from a certain part of the world, I like to put on music from that culture and pretend that I am there. That is why I wanted this book to feature easy recipes from all over the world.

I hope you have fun with this book and can pretend you are in all the different places each dish is from. Bon Appetit!

CONTENTS

117 Asia and the Pacific

157 Index

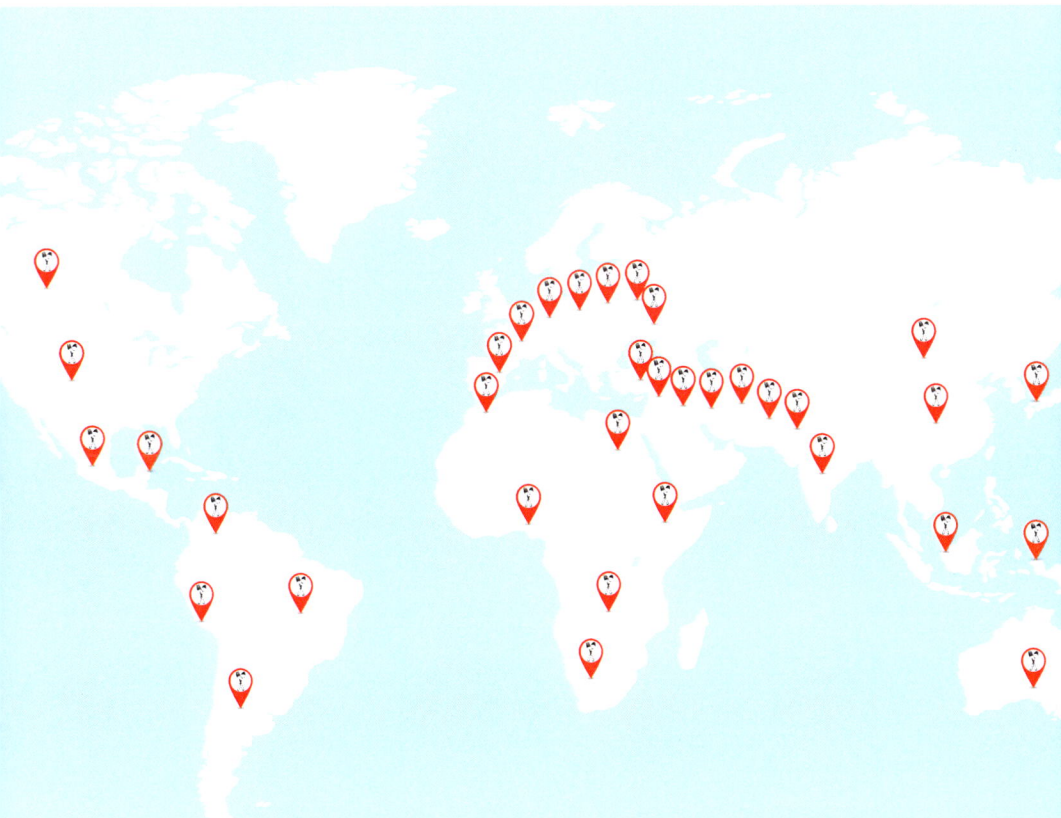

HOW TO USE THIS BOOK

This book is designed to take you across the world with your taste buds. I have organized the book into three regions: The Americas; Europe, Africa, and the Middle East; and Asia/Pacific. We even have a recipe from Antarctica!

Each section features dinner, lunch, and breakfast recipes from that region, and many of them have been modified so they are easier to cook. Some of the recipes have specific notes at the bottom indicating how they are accessible to a variety of people, which was very important to me.

Occasionally, a recipe has some optional ingredients or ways you can switch things up based on personal preference. I believe that experimentation while cooking is key to learning how to be a good chef. I also have a list of all the major tools you will need for each recipe to make it easier for you to have everything set out and ready to go before you start cooking.

If you are new to cooking, my recommendation is to try and taste everything before you serve it, so you can start to learn how certain spices and ingredients work together. Don't be afraid to really jump into cooking and find a few dishes that you really enjoy making and sharing with others. Even if you can't travel the world, my hope is that with this book you can experience all the wonderful flavors out there.

IMPORTANT COOKING TIPS AND TOOLS

Whether you are a professionally trained chef or just learning how to boil water, having the right tools is a non-negotiable. Similarly, there are some tried and true rules of cooking that are good to know so you can build a solid foundation and, most importantly, stay safe while in the kitchen.

Here are some basic kitchen "rules" to keep in mind:

Never leave a hot stove unattended. It may seem like it will only take a couple of minutes to answer the door or take the dog outside, but it takes only a few seconds for a boiling-over pot to become a big problem. If you have to leave the stove area for anything, simply turn off the burners and turn them back on when you return.

Know your proper cooking temperatures for meat (and eggs). Not all types of animal proteins need to be cooked to the same temperature, and even a few degrees below the minimum threshold for cooked meat can pose a health risk. Here's a simple primer: eggs and ground meats should be cooked to 160 degrees Fahrenheit; poultry and other water fowl to 165 degrees Fahrenheit; and steaks/chops/roasts should be cooked to 145 degrees Fahrenheit.

Always use heat-resistant gloves when using the oven. You may think you can just quickly move that dish or stir that bubbling casserole without wearing gloves, but remember that the entire inside of the oven is hot, and an oven burn is a real quick way to ruin your meal…and your day!

Read a recipe all the way through before you begin. Reading a recipe all the way through is a good way to make sure you not only have all the ingredients you need, but you have all of the right tools as well. Try and have all your ingredients and tools set out before you begin working, so you aren't running to the pantry or fridge in the middle of a crucial step in the recipe.

Taste and season as you go. Not only does this ensure a balanced flavor, but it also teaches you about ingredients and spices each time you cook. Before you know it, you'll be a master chef!

And here are some basic kitchen tools to have on hand:

Every chef is only as good as their best knife. It's true, and quality tools can elevate the whole experience of creating a meal.

But that doesn't mean you need to break the bank buying all the trendy cooking appliances you see on TV. Here are the 10 tools you will need for the recipes in this book, and having these basic tools will make it possible for you to make many other meals as well.

A large skillet. A cast-iron skillet is the industry standard - and for good reason - but any non-stick skillet will work. Treat your skillet well. If it's cast iron, avoid getting it super wet, and if you need to clean it make sure you dry it thoroughly afterwards (many people even dry theirs over a warm stove) and lightly "season" it with oil to prevent rusting.

Basic 5-piece cooking utensil set (plus a few more). You can use any utensil brand, but wooden spoons are preferred because they last forever. The five-piece set includes a large spoon, spatula, scraper, server, and tongs. Add in a whisk, a handheld grater, and a slotted spoon and you're all set.

Large and small pots. You only need one large and one small pot for sauces and soups, but having a couple more on hand is good if you have a recipe where maybe you need to be cooking more than one thing at a time over the stove. Yes, it means you'll have to clean something else, but trust me…it's worth it.

Baking dishes and sheets. Again, you might only need one large glass dish and one small one, but having a variety of sizes makes it possible to cook more than one thing at a time, and to also double or triple a recipe for a large crowd. A glass baking dish is deep, whereas a baking sheet (think what you bake cookies on) is flat and sometimes slightly curved around the edges.

Sharp knives. How many knives do you need? As many as you want! Well, a good place to start is with a knife set in a wooden butcher block.

These sets typically include one versatile chef's knife, a serrated knife, a paring knife, a utility knife, and usually some kitchen shears. Knives can be expensive, but they are an investment, and one you usually only buy once. Get them sharpened regularly for longevity and effectiveness.

Colander. A lot of the recipes in my book require a colander to rinse cooked pasta or vegetables. A steel colander will last you forever, but you might also want to get a mesh one if you are rinsing rice or something else with very small pieces.

Slow cooker and Instant Pot. There is nothing quite like slow-cooked meat; it's tender, juicy, and worth the wait. They are also great for meal preparation because you can throw everything inside the pot in the morning and have dinner waiting for you later in the day. Instant Pots often feature slow cooker settings, so I would recommend splurging for one Instant Pot rather than a slow cooker and an Instant Pot. Best of all, Instant Pots can be used to make a variety of things, from soups and meats to yogurt and desserts!

Blender. Yes, blenders are great for morning smoothies, but they are also very useful for making desserts, sauces, and even pureeing vegetables. You don't need a fancy one, but try to get one that has a few speed options.

Measuring cups and spoons. Don't try to eyeball that tablespoon of fish sauce! Have on hand a full set of measuring cups and spoons ranging from the tiniest ¼ teaspoon all the way to one full cup. Many of these sets come linked together, so you can easily keep track of them in a kitchen drawer and pull them out when needed.

Meat thermometer. As I mentioned earlier, cooking meat and eggs to the right temperature doesn't just equal good taste; it also ensures food safety. Having a food thermometer takes all the guesswork out of it.

The Americas

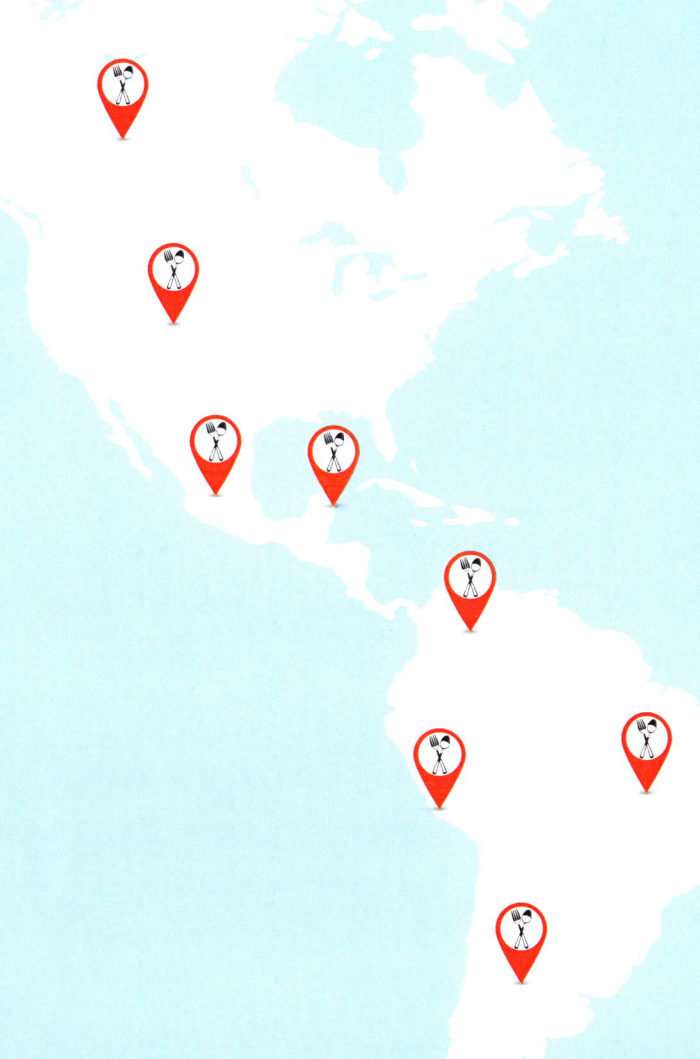

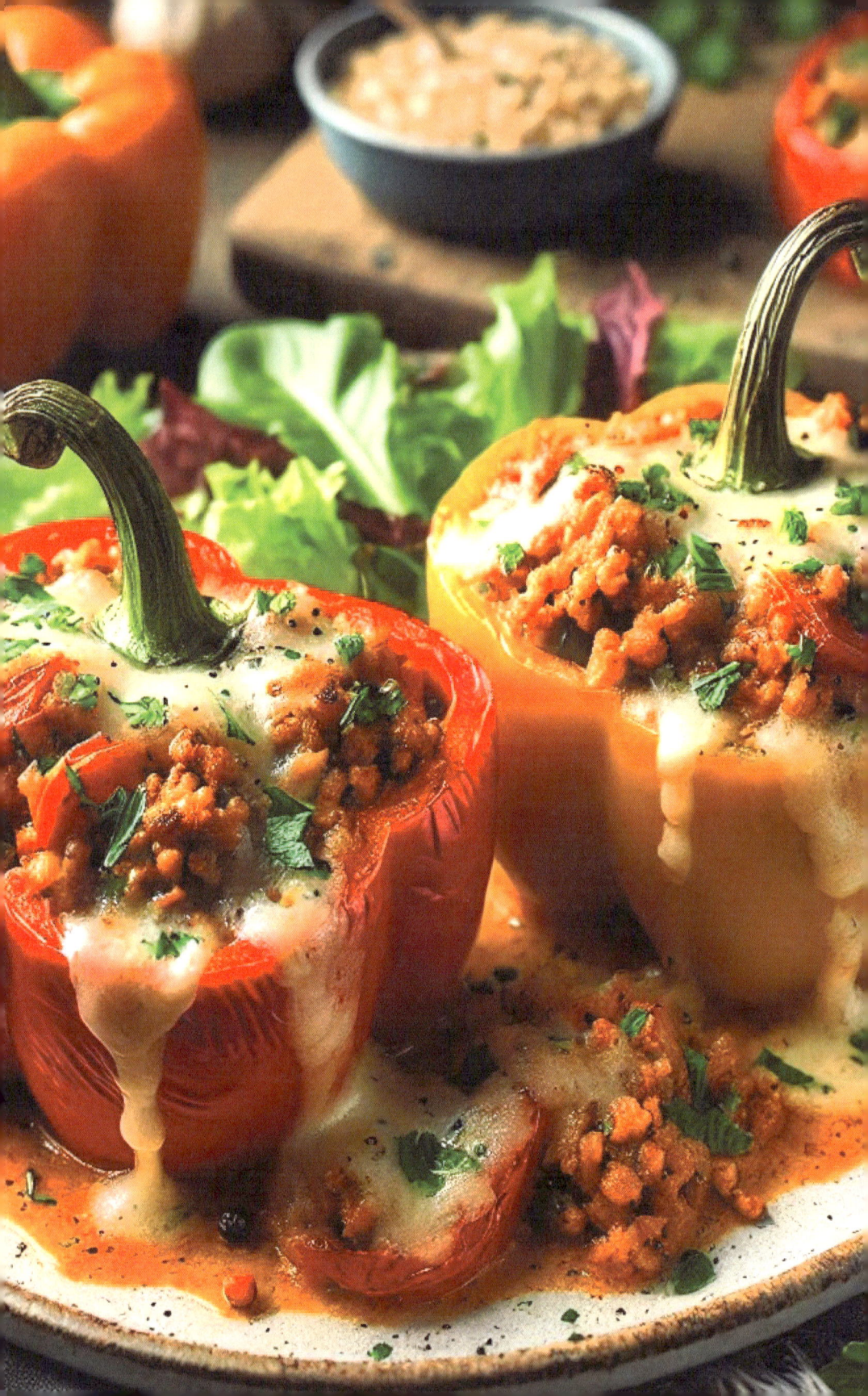

American Stuffed Peppers

Stuffed peppers are a great way to get some good veggies in your diet. I like to top mine with some cheddar cheese and let it melt on top before serving, but you can keep this dairy-free or even make it vegetarian by using crumbled tempeh instead of ground beef.

Ingredients:

1 pound of ground beef
3 bell peppers (red, yellow, or orange)
1 tablespoon olive oil
1 tablespoon tomato paste
2 garlic cloves (minced)
1 small onion (chopped)
Salt and pepper to taste
Optional: ½ cup shredded cheddar cheese
for topping

Tools You'll Need:

Medium skillet or frying pan
Baking sheet or glass dish
Measuring cups and spoons
Spatula or wooden spoon
Small bowl

Step-by-Step Instructions:

1 Cook your meat and onion.
Add your oil to the skillet and heat on medium until not quite smoking, then add garlic and sauté for one minute until fragrant. Add onion and cook until it softens, 2 to 3 minutes. Add your ground beef, and season with some salt and pepper, breaking up the meat with a spatula or wooden spoon as it cooks. Cook for 8-10 minutes until no longer pink.

2 Heat your oven to 350 degrees F and prepare your pepper cups.
Wash your peppers, cut off the top of them, and remove any seeds inside. Lightly grease your baking dish or add aluminum foil to a baking sheet and place the peppers on top, then use a spoon to fill each one with your cooked beef.

3 Bake your stuffed peppers.
Bake your peppers for 20 minutes. Remove and sprinkle cheese on immediately so it melts on top, or place back in the oven and broil for 1-2 minutes until golden brown. Serve alongside rice or salad.

Arepa Pizza Bites

In Venezuela, arepas are a common street food and are usually topped with cheese. This fun twist on the arepa makes them into little cornmeal pizzas. They are easy to put together and fun to eat.

Ingredients:
(Makes 4 mini pizzas)
1 cup pre-cooked white cornmeal (Harina P.A.N. – common in Venezuelan cooking)
1 ¼ cups warm water
½ tsp salt
1 tbsp vegetable oil (for cooking)
½ cup shredded cheese (mozzarella or any favorite)
1 small tomato (chopped)
1 boiled egg (chopped)
1 tbsp ketchup or tomato sauce
A pinch of oregano (optional)

Tools You'll Need:
A mixing bowl
A spoon
A non-stick frying pan or griddle
A spatula
A butter knife or spoon for spreading

Step-by-Step Instructions:

1 Make the Dough
In a bowl, mix the warm water and salt. Slowly add the cornmeal while mixing with a spoon or clean hands until it feels like soft Play-Doh. Let it rest for 2 minutes.

2 Shape the Arepa Discs
Divide the dough into 4 equal balls. Flatten each ball into a small, round patty—like a thick mini pizza crust (about the size of your palm).

3 Cook the Arepas
Heat the pan over medium heat and add a little oil. Cook each arepa for 4-5 minutes on each side, until lightly golden and firm to the touch.

4 Top Your Arepas
Turn off the heat. Spread a little ketchup or tomato sauce on top of each arepa. Add cheese, chopped tomato, and boiled egg on top like mini pizzas. Sprinkle a little oregano if you'd like!

5 Melt & Serve
If you want the cheese melted, cover the pan for 1 minute. Then remove from heat and let cool slightly. Serve warm and enjoy your Arepa Pizza Bites!

Tips for Accessibility:
Use pre-boiled eggs or boil them the night before.
All toppings can be prepared in advance.
Encourage creativity: Try avocado slices or ham as toppings!

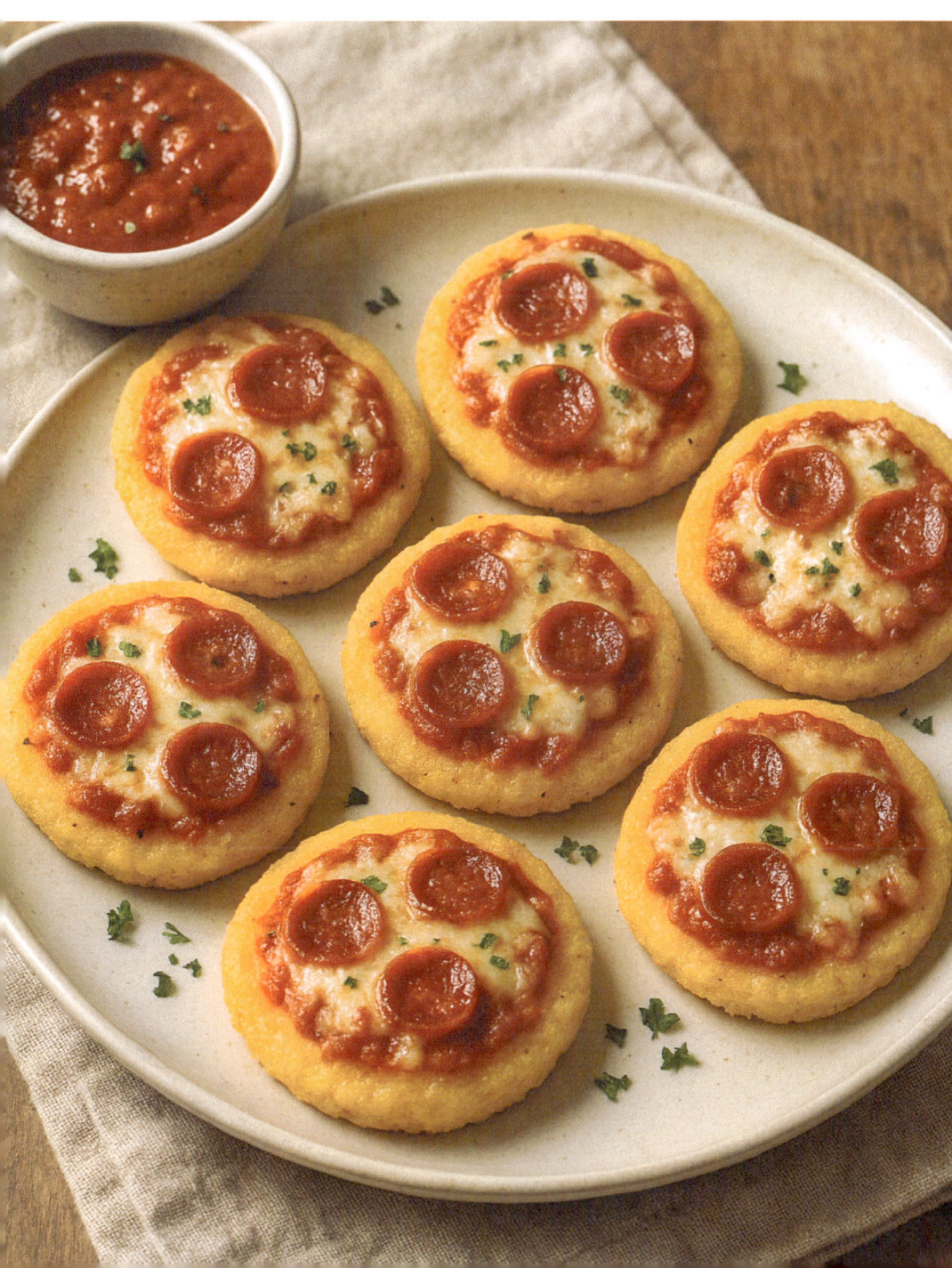

Argentinian Matambre

In Spanish, "Matar Hambre" means to cut hunger, which is what this quick cooking cut of steak (the flank steak) is known for. This South American dish is surprisingly easy to come together. If you don't know how to butterfly cut your flank steak, have the butcher do it ahead of time.

Ingredients:

2 lbs. flank steak
¼ cup Olive Oil + 1 Tbsp for cooking peppers
4 cloves garlic (minced)
¼ cup cilantro (chopped)
¼ cup parsley (chopped)
1 tablespoon salt
1 tablespoon pepper
1 tablespoon red pepper flakes
4 hard-boiled eggs (peeled and cut into quarters)
½ green bell pepper (sliced into strips)
½ red bell pepper (sliced into strips)
2 carrots (thinly sliced)

Tools You'll Need:

Baking sheet
Aluminum foil
Measuring cups and spoons
Cutting Board
Plastic wrap
Sharp knife
Meat pounder *(Not a meat tenderizer – make sure it doesn't have teeth.)*
Mixing bowl
Paper-towel-lined plate
Small skillet and spatula or tongs
Cooking twine

Step-by-Step Instructions:

1 Preheat your oven to 350 degrees.
  Line a baking sheet with aluminum foil.

2 Butterfly cut your steak.
  Towel dry your steak and lay it flat on a cutting board. Starting at one of the shorter ends, cut through the flank steak going almost to the other end. Now, open up the meat so it lays like an open book. Place a piece of plastic food film over the meat. Using a meat pounder, pound the meat so that it evens out.

3 Make your chimichurri sauce.
  In a small bowl mix together your olive oil, garlic, parsley, cilantro, salt, pepper and red pepper flakes. Set aside.

4 Sauté your peppers and carrots.
  Add the remaining tablespoon of olive oil to a small skillet and heat on medium-high heat. Add sliced bell peppers and carrots and sauté until soft. Remove from the pan and place on a paper-towel-lined plate to soak up the extra oil.

5 Assemble your flank steak rolls.
  Spread the chimichurri mixture on butterfly-cut flank steak. Next, arrange pieces

of hard-boiled eggs on top, followed by the pepper and carrot mixture. Gently roll flank steak up starting from the shortest end (like a jelly roll) and tie with pieces of cooking twine so it is tightly together. Set on baking sheet.

6 Bake at 350 degrees for one hour.
Remove from the oven and let sit for 15 minutes before slicing and then serving.

Tips for Accessibility:

Find a pre-cut flank steak and ask a butcher to cut it for you.

Fill the roll with store-bought chimichurri sauce rather than making your own.

Use store-bought hard-boiled eggs.

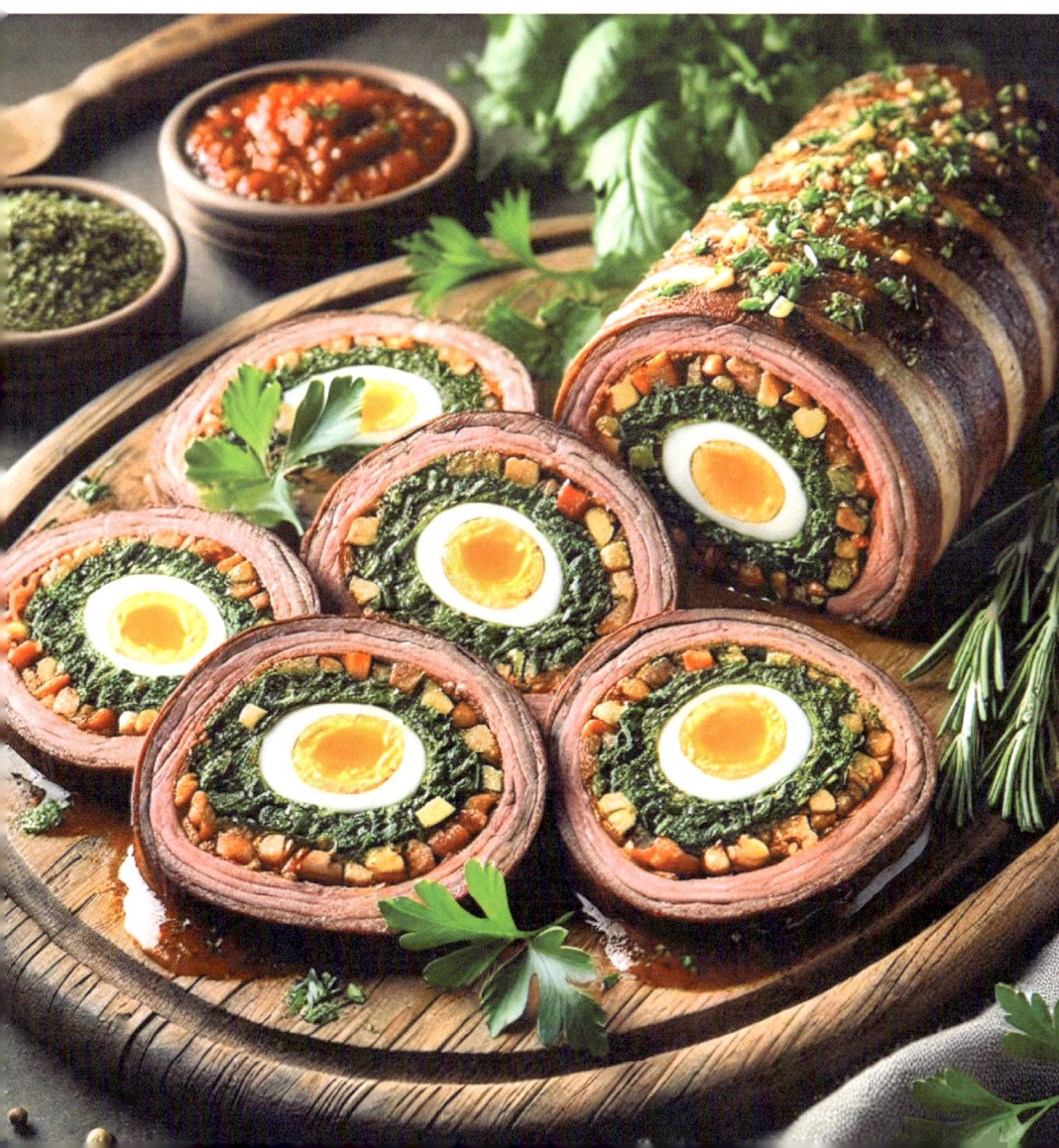

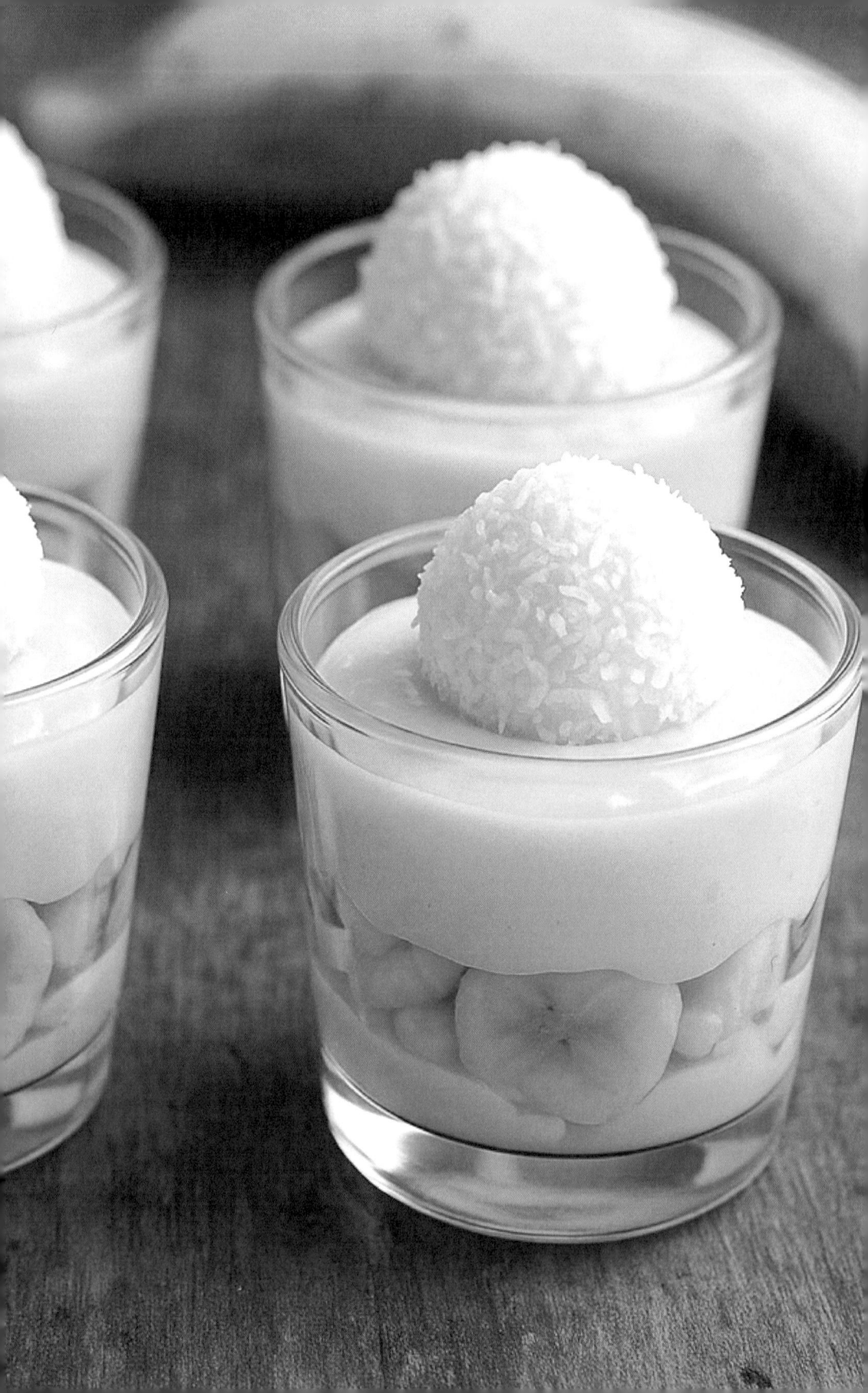

Banana Beijinho Cups

A tropical twist on Brazil's classic "beijinho" (little coconut truffle), layered in a cup with banana slices for a creamy, fruity treat!

Ingredients:
(Makes 4 small cups)
1 can sweetened condensed milk (14 oz)
1 tablespoon butter
½ cup shredded coconut (unsweetened or sweetened)
1 ripe banana (sliced into coins)
Extra shredded coconut or sprinkles for topping
4 small paper or plastic cups

Tools You'll Need:
Small saucepan
Spoon or spatula
Stove or hot plate (with supervision)
Butter knife (for slicing banana)
Small cups or bowls

Step-by-Step Instructions:

1 Make the coconut cream.
   In a small pan, add the butter and condensed milk. Stir on low heat for 5–8 minutes until it gets thick like pudding. Stir in the shredded coconut. Let it cool for 10 minutes.

2 Slice the banana.
   Use a butter knife to slice the banana into small, round pieces.

3 Assemble the cups.
   In each cup, place a few banana slices on the bottom. Add 2 spoonfuls of the coconut cream on top. Then a few more banana slices, and finish with another spoon of coconut cream.

4 Top and chill.
   Sprinkle with a little extra coconut or colorful sprinkles. Chill in the fridge for 10–15 minutes (or just eat it soft and warm!).

Tips for Accessibility:
You can make the coconut cream ahead of time and store it in the fridge.

Instead of cooking, you can also mix sweetened condensed milk with coconut straight from the can for a no-cook version—just keep it refrigerated.

The cups can be layered however you like—no wrong way!

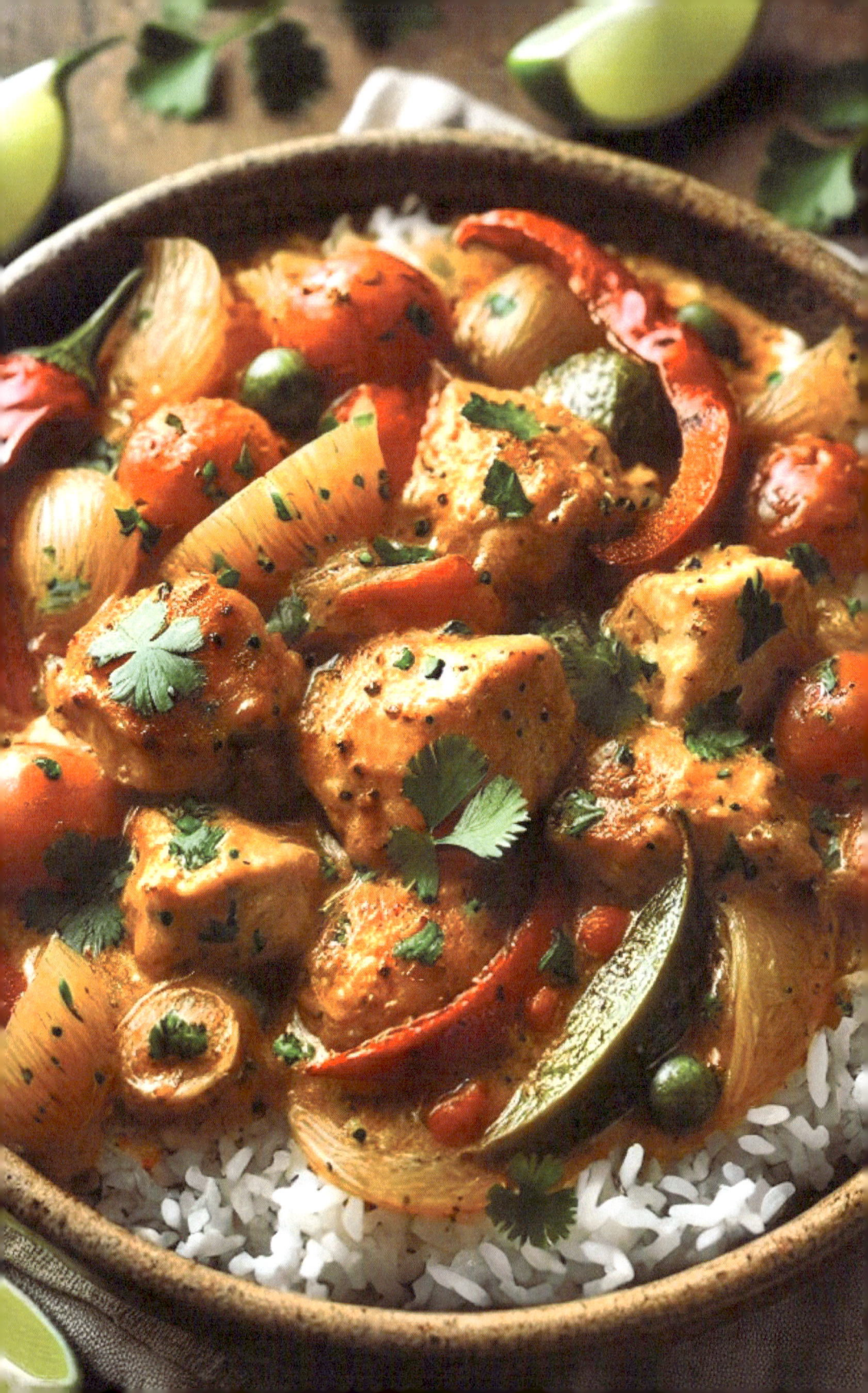

Brazilian Spicy Coconut Chicken

This spicy dish is popular in Brazil and is a good meal to double the recipe so you can eat it all week. If you don't like spicy foods, simply omit the jalapeño peppers and/or cayenne pepper. This dish is delicious served over rice, quinoa, or try dipping some fresh bread in the sauce.

Ingredients:

4 skinless, boneless chicken breasts cut in half
1 14 oz. can of light coconut milk
3 chopped tomatoes (or 1 small can diced tomatoes)
1 diced jalapeño pepper
2 tablespoons olive oil, halved
1 chopped white onion
½ cup shredded, unsweetened coconut
2 cloves minced garlic
2 tablespoon minced fresh ginger
1 teaspoon ground cumin
1 teaspoon ground cayenne pepper
1 teaspoon ground turmeric
1 teaspoon ground coriander
Salt and pepper to taste

Tools You'll Need:

Large skillet
Measuring cups and spoons
Plate and paper towels

Tips for Accessibility:

Use canned tomatoes for less cutting.

Omit any spicy ingredients (cayenne and jalapeño) if desired.

Coconut milk is poured straight from a can—no prep.

Step-by-Step Instructions:

1 Cook chicken.
   Heat 1 tablespoon olive oil in a skillet over medium heat. Place chicken breasts in the skillet and cook 7-12 minutes on each side until done and juices run clear. Remove from heat and set aside on a plate lined with paper towels.

2 Make your spicy coconut sauce.
   Heat the remaining tablespoon of olive oil in the skillet on medium heat. Cook the onion, ginger, jalapeño, and garlic for about 5 minutes, stirring occasionally, until tender. Add in the tomatoes and cook for an additional 5 to 8 minutes. Stir in the coconut milk and shredded coconut and continue to stir until all ingredients are mixed and heated through.

3 Plate your chicken and pour your sauce on top.
   This is best served over rice, but you can eat it on its own as well.

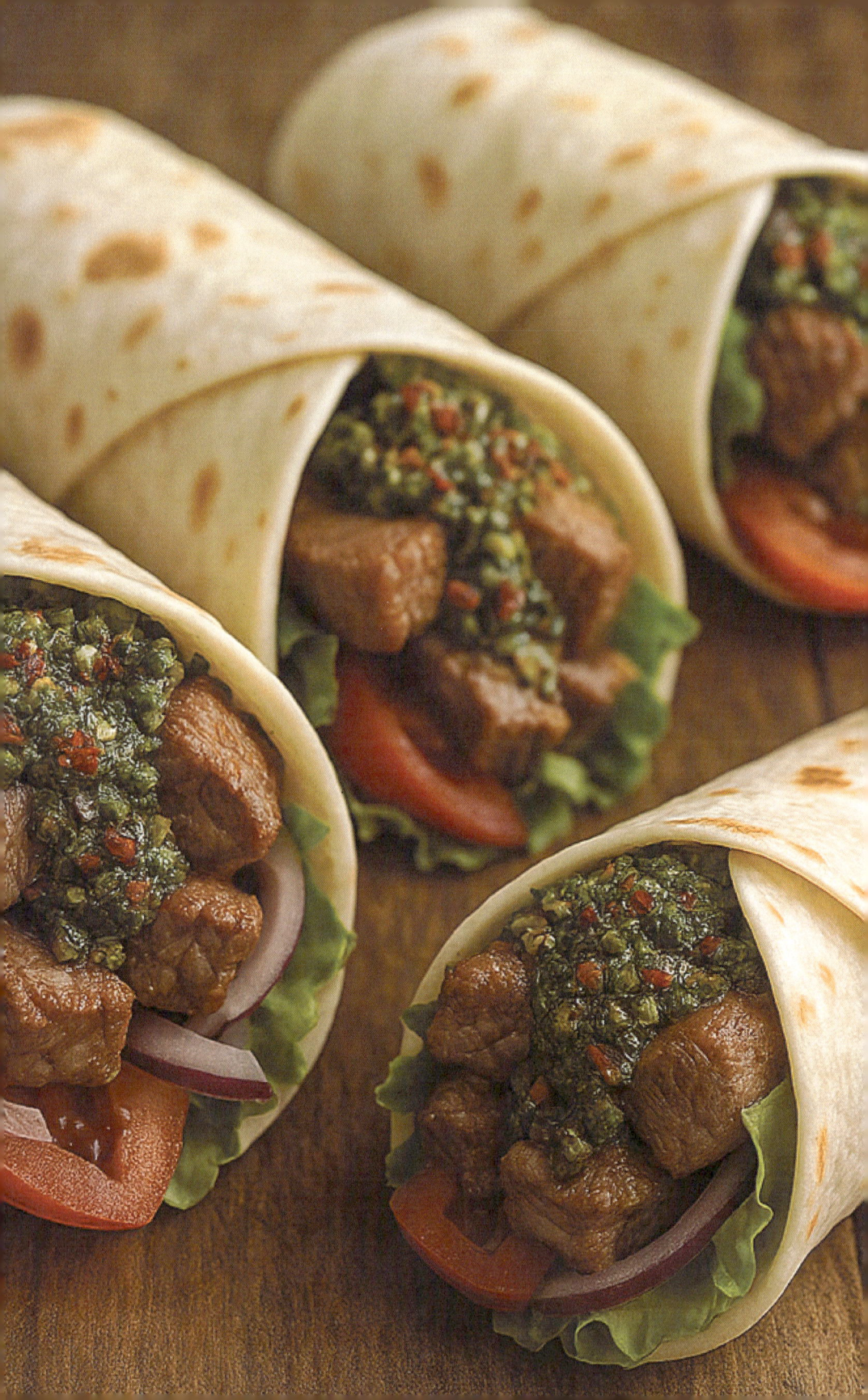

Argentine Beef & Chimichurri Wraps

A warm tortilla filled with seasoned beef, soft vegetables, and a simple chimichurri-inspired sauce. This recipe is a great way to use leftover ground beef, and feel free just to use store-bought chimichurri to save you even more time.

Ingredients:
(Makes 2 wraps)
½ cup cooked ground beef (or shredded chicken or lentils)
2 small flour tortillas (or corn if preferred)
¼ cup cooked or canned chopped carrots (or bell peppers)
2 tablespoons shredded cheese (mozzarella or cheddar)
1 tablespoon oil or butter

For the chimichurri sauce:
2 tablespoons plain yogurt or sour cream
1 teaspoon dried parsley (or fresh)
½ teaspoon vinegar or lemon juice
A pinch of garlic powder and salt

Step-by-Step Instructions:

1 Heat the filling.
In a pan, warm the cooked ground beef and carrots with a tiny bit of oil (or microwave for 1–2 minutes). Sprinkle cheese on top to melt.

2 Make the Chimichurri sauce.
In a small bowl, mix yogurt, parsley, vinegar, garlic powder, and a pinch of salt. Stir with a spoon.

3 Warm the tortillas.
Warm each tortilla in the microwave for 15 seconds to make them soft and bendy.

4 Assemble the wrap.
Place warm beef and veggie mix in the center of each tortilla. Drizzle with chimichurri sauce. Fold up the bottom, then fold the sides over to make a wrap.

5 Eat and enjoy.
Serve warm with a napkin. Easy to hold and eat by hand or cut in half.

Tools You'll Need:
Frying pan or microwave
Spoon
Small bowl
Plate

Tips for Accessibility:
Use pre-cooked or leftover beef to avoid raw handling.

All ingredients are soft and spoonable.

Yogurt sauce adds color and flavor without needing a blender or sharp tools.

Tortillas are easier than empañada dough—no sealing or baking!

Visual cues help with folding steps (fold up the bottom, then the sides).

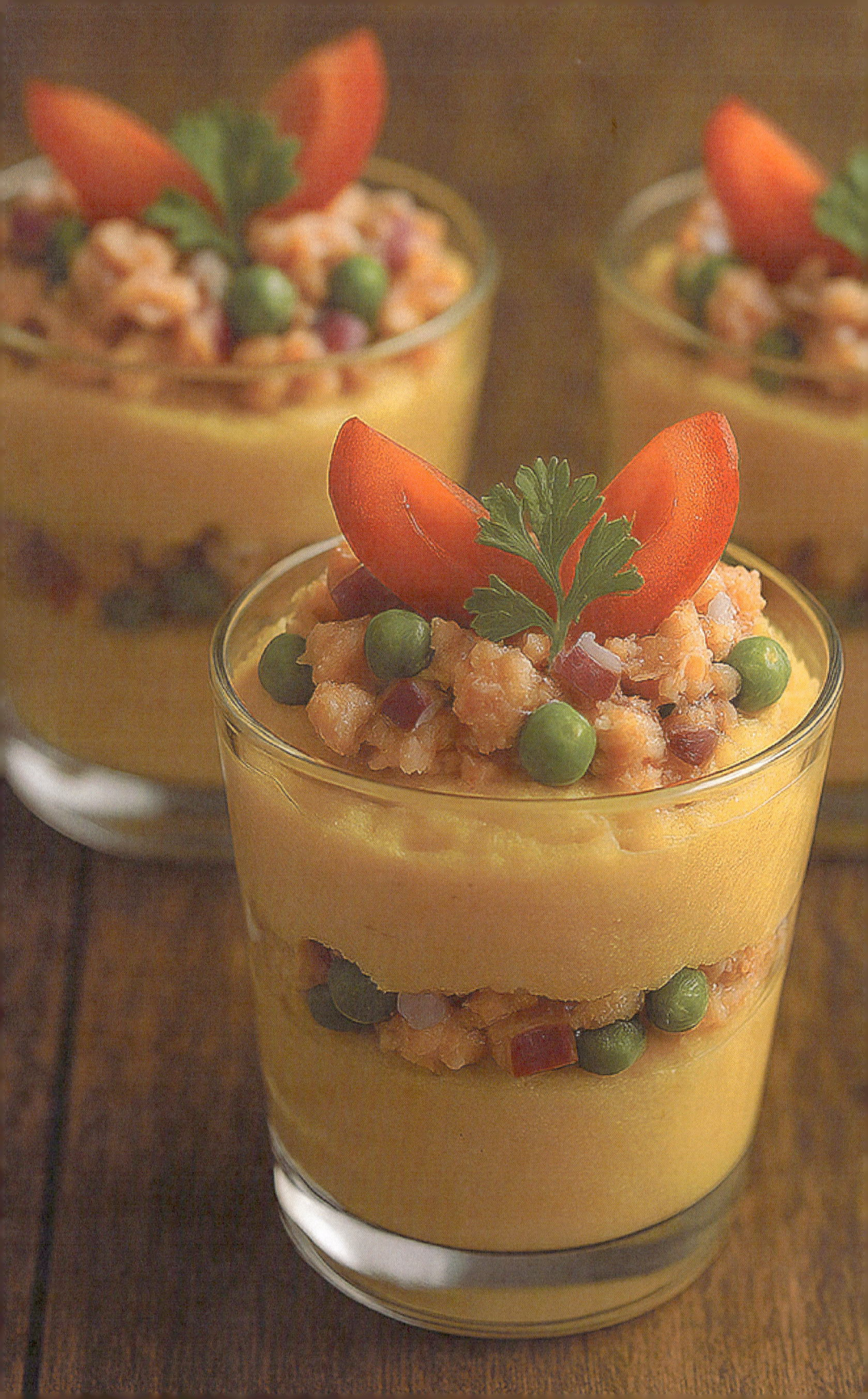

Causa Lunch Cups

A soft and creamy Peruvian potato and avocado lunch served in a cup—layered, colorful, and no stove or knives needed!

Ingredients:
(Makes 2–3 small cups)
1 ½ cups instant mashed potatoes (prepared and cooled)
1 small can of tuna or shredded rotisserie chicken (drained)
1 tablespoon mayonnaise
½ ripe avocado (mashed with a fork)
1 tablespoon lime juice (optional)
Salt to taste
Optional: 1 tablespoon cooked carrots or peas (for color)

Tools You'll Need:
Bowl and spoon
Fork
2–3 small clear cups or bowls for layering

Step-by-Step Instructions:

1 Prepare the fillings.
   In a bowl, mix the tuna (or chicken) with mayo. In another small bowl, mash the avocado with a fork and stir in lime juice if using. Add a pinch of salt to both.

2 Layer the cups.
   In each cup, add a spoonful of mashed potato, then a layer of avocado, then a layer of the tuna or chicken. Repeat layers if you have more space.

3 Add color (Optional).
   Sprinkle a few peas or chopped cooked carrots on top for a colorful finish.

4 Chill or eat.
   You can eat it right away or chill it for 10–15 minutes. Eat with a spoon—no cutting needed!

Tips for Accessibility:
Use instant mashed potatoes to avoid peeling and boiling.
Canned tuna or rotisserie chicken requires no cooking.
Fork-mashing and spoon-layering are safe and tactile steps.
Bright colors and layers make it fun and visually rewarding.
Everything is soft and scoopable with a spoon.

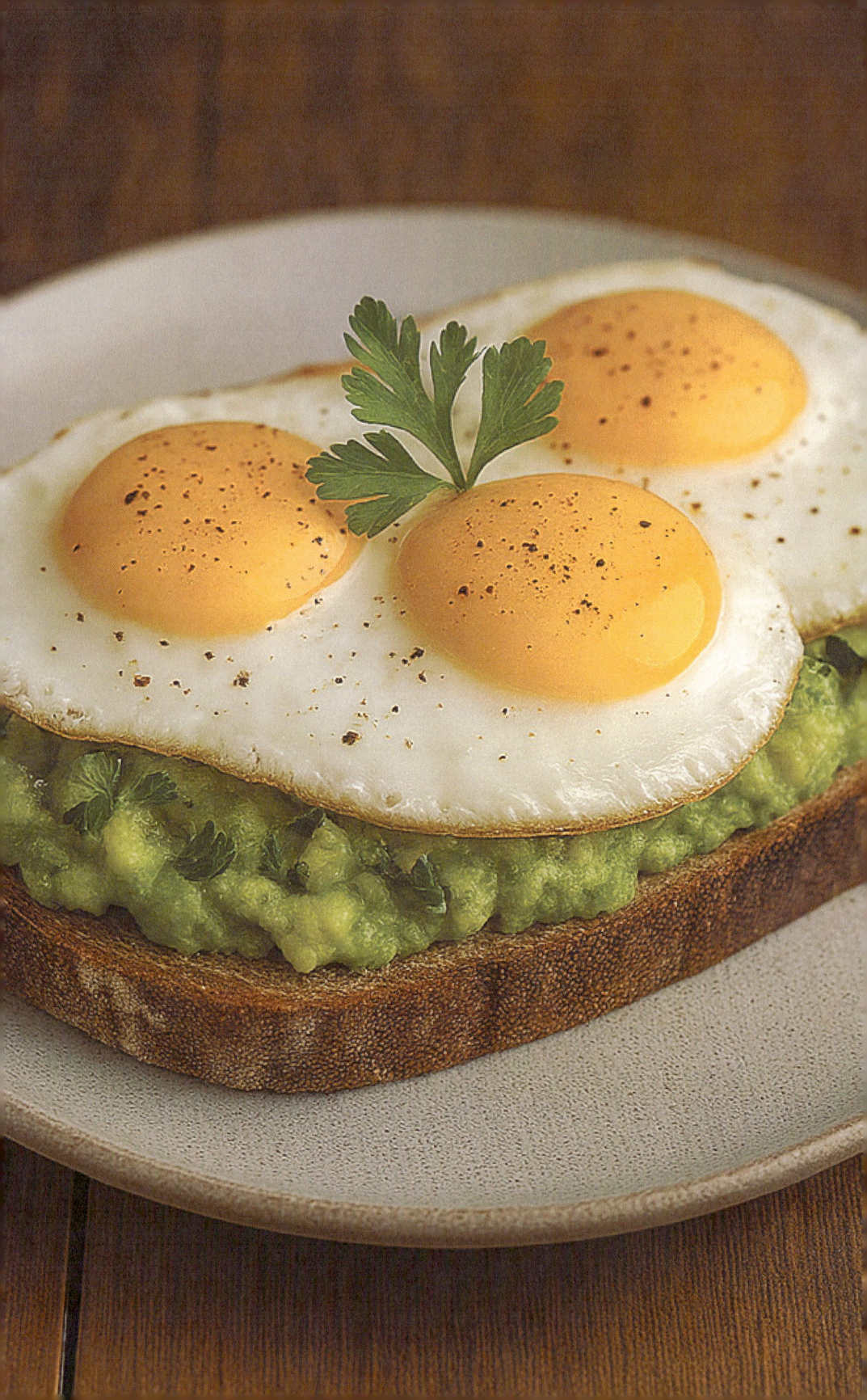

Chilean Pan con Palta y Huevo

Bread with avocado and egg – a classic Chilean breakfast made simple!

Ingredients:
(Makes 2 pieces)
2 slices of marraqueta or any soft bread roll (or use regular sliced bread)
1 ripe avocado
2 eggs
½ teaspoon lemon juice (optional, to keep avocado green)
A pinch of salt
A tiny bit of oil or butter (for cooking)

Tools You'll Need:
Fork
Bowl
Frying pan
Spatula
Toaster or pan to warm the bread

Step-by-Step Instructions:

1 **Mash the avocado.**
Cut the avocado in half (get help if needed), scoop out the green part into a bowl, and mash it with a fork. Add lemon juice and a pinch of salt. Mix and set aside.

2 **Cook the eggs.**
Put a tiny bit of oil or butter in the pan. Heat on medium.
Crack one egg into the pan. Cook it how you like:
  Scrambled: stir with a spatula
  Fried: leave it whole and cook both sides
  Repeat for the second egg. Then turn off the heat.

3 **Toast the bread.**
Warm the bread in a toaster or in the oven for 1–2 minutes.

4 **Assemble your avocado on toast.**
Spread mashed avocado on each piece of bread. Place one cooked egg on top of each. Sprinkle with a little more salt if you like.

5 **Eat and enjoy.**
Serve warm, with a napkin or on a plate. Easy to eat with your hands or a fork!

Tips for Accessibility:
Use pre-mashed avocado or avocado spread if cutting is difficult.

Bread can be warmed in the microwave instead of a pan.

Practice egg-cracking using a bowl with a wide rim or use a pourable egg substitute.

Safe with minimal tools and just one pan.

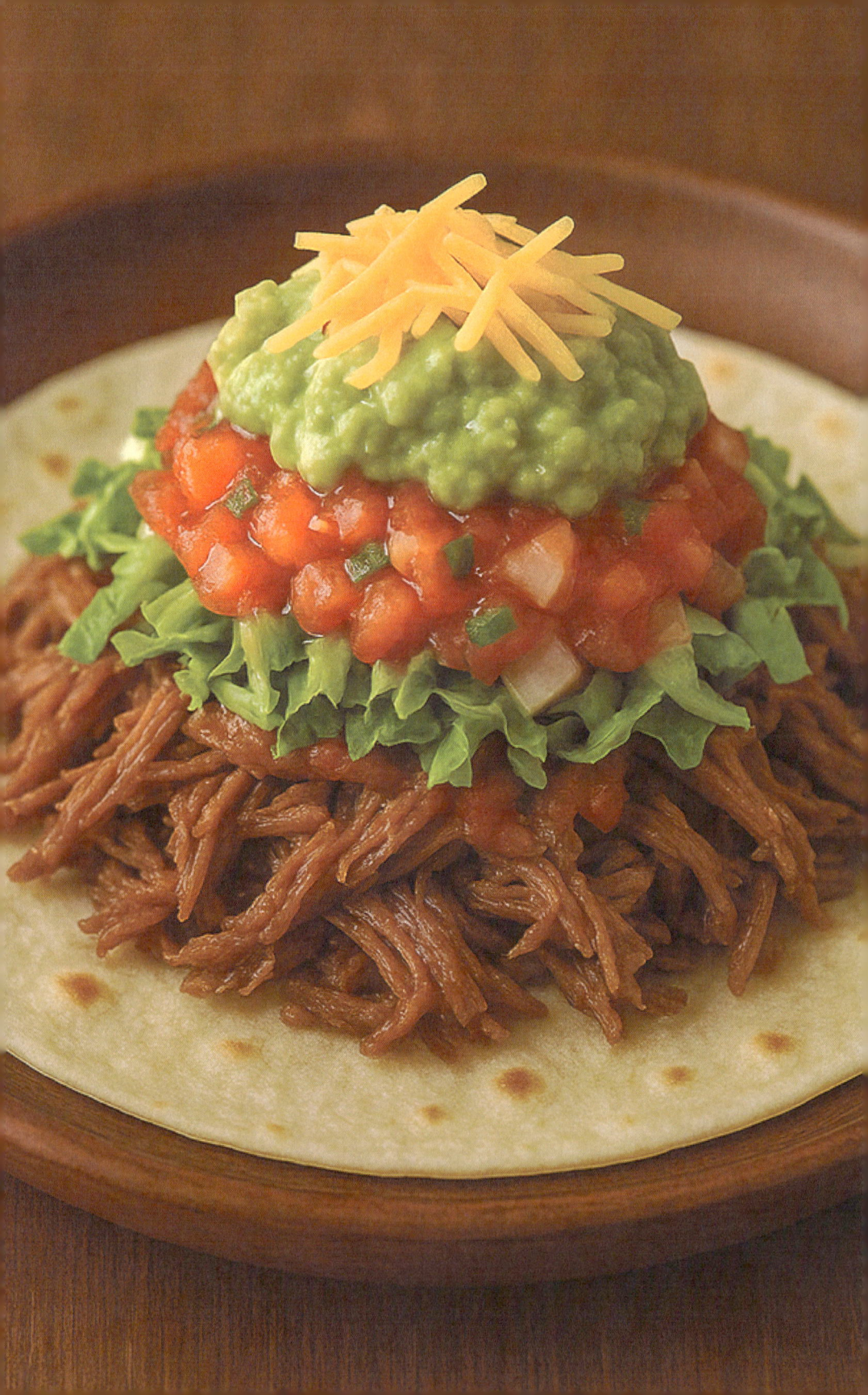

Crop Top Cuban Pork

Pork is extremely flavorful when cooked in a slow cooker. Slow cooker recipes like this one are great for busy days because you can toss the ingredients in the pot in the morning and then let it cook during the day, so it's ready when you walk in the door. I like to eat this pork in tortillas, similar to a taco, but you can also serve it over rice or vegetables and create a bowl with what you have on hand.

Ingredients:
3-pound pork shoulder roast
½ cup lemon juice
¼ cup water
¼ cup tomato sauce
¼ cup tomato paste
1 cup chopped onion
3 cloves minced garlic
3 bay leaves
1 teaspoon dried oregano
½ teaspoon ground cumin
½ teaspoon salt
¼ teaspoon black pepper

Tools You'll Need:
Crockpot (or InstaPot with a slow cooker setting)
Measuring cups and spoons
Cutting board
Knife
Cooking Tongs
Two forks

Step-by-Step Instructions:

1 Add all ingredients to your slow cooker.
Cook on HIGH for six hours.

2 Shred pork.
Carefully remove the meat using kitchen tongs to a cutting board, shred the pork using two forks, and place it in a large serving platter.

3 Serve with desired toppings/sides.
Try whole wheat tortillas, salsa, lettuce, guacamole, and shredded cheese for tacos.

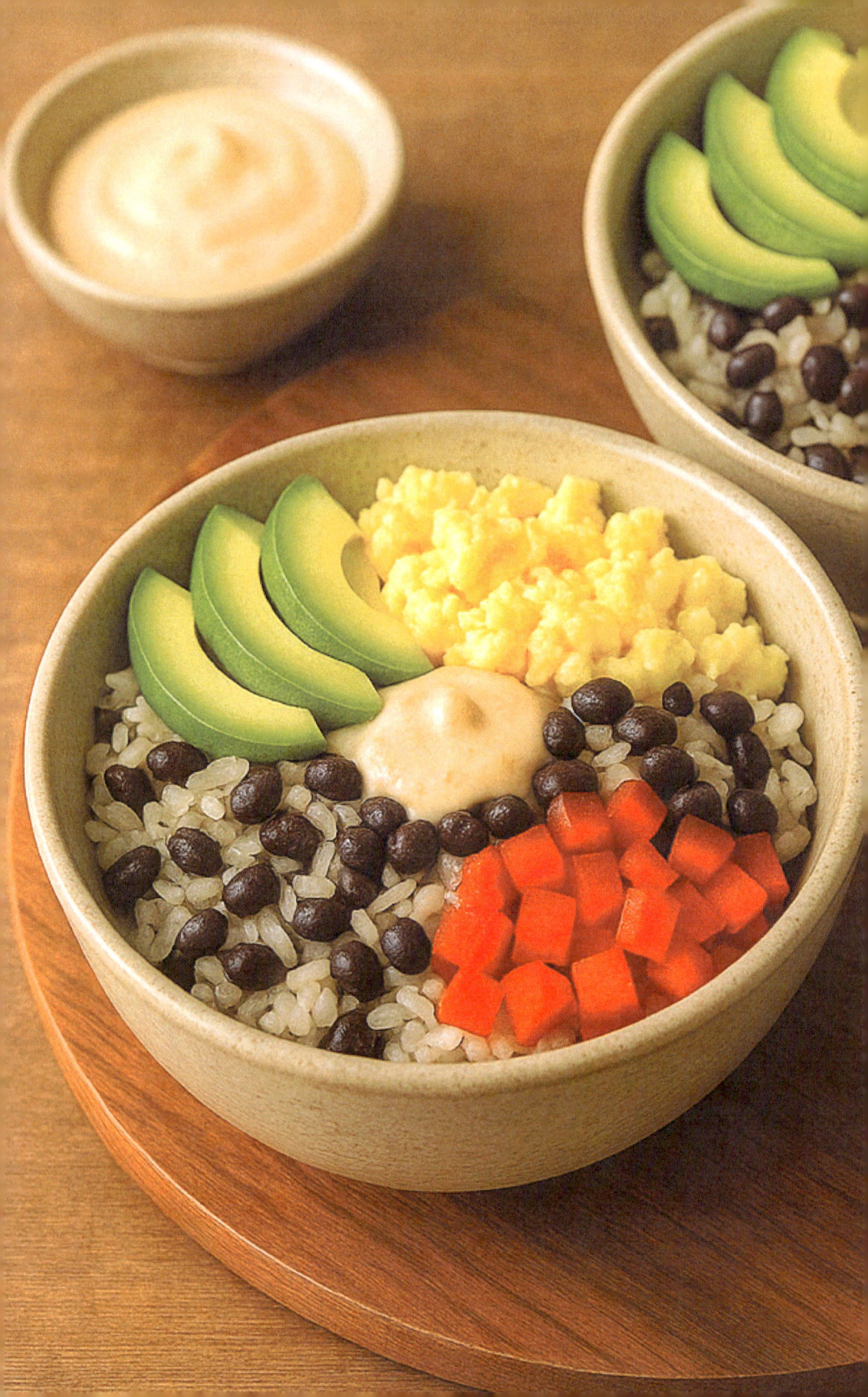

Gallo Pinto Lunch Bowls

A warm, soft Nicaraguan-style rice and beans bowl with gentle seasoning and optional sweet plantains—flavorful, filling, and fun to eat!

Ingredients:
(Makes 2 servings)
1 cup cooked white rice (microwaveable or leftover)
½ cup canned black beans (drained and rinsed)
2 tablespoons onion flakes (or pre-chopped onion, optional)
1 tablespoon oil or butter
½ teaspoon ground cumin
A pinch of salt
Optional: 1 small banana or sweet plantain, sliced and microwaved
Optional: 2 tablespoons sour cream or plain yogurt for topping

Tools You'll Need:
Frying pan or microwave-safe bowl
Spoon
Serving bowl or plate

Tips for Accessibility:
Microwave rice and canned beans reduce steps and heat risk.

No chopping needed—onion flakes add flavor safely.

Bananas are easy to slice with a butter knife and microwave.

Only one pan or bowl needed—minimal cleanup.

Soft, colorful, and familiar ingredients help with confidence and independence.

Step-by-Step Instructions:

1 Warm the base.
Heat oil in a pan over medium heat (or use a microwave-safe bowl with oil). Add onion flakes, rice, and beans. Stir gently.

2 Add seasoning.
Sprinkle in cumin and a pinch of salt. Stir everything together and cook for about 5 minutes (or microwave for 2–3 minutes) until warm and blended.

3 Prepare the plantains or bananas.(Optional)
Place banana or sweet plantain slices on a plate. Microwave for 1 minute until soft and warm.

4 Assemble the bowl.
Spoon the rice and beans into a bowl. Add the soft banana slices on the side. Top with a spoonful of sour cream or yogurt if you like.

5 Serve and enjoy.
Eat warm with a spoon. All textures are soft and comforting!

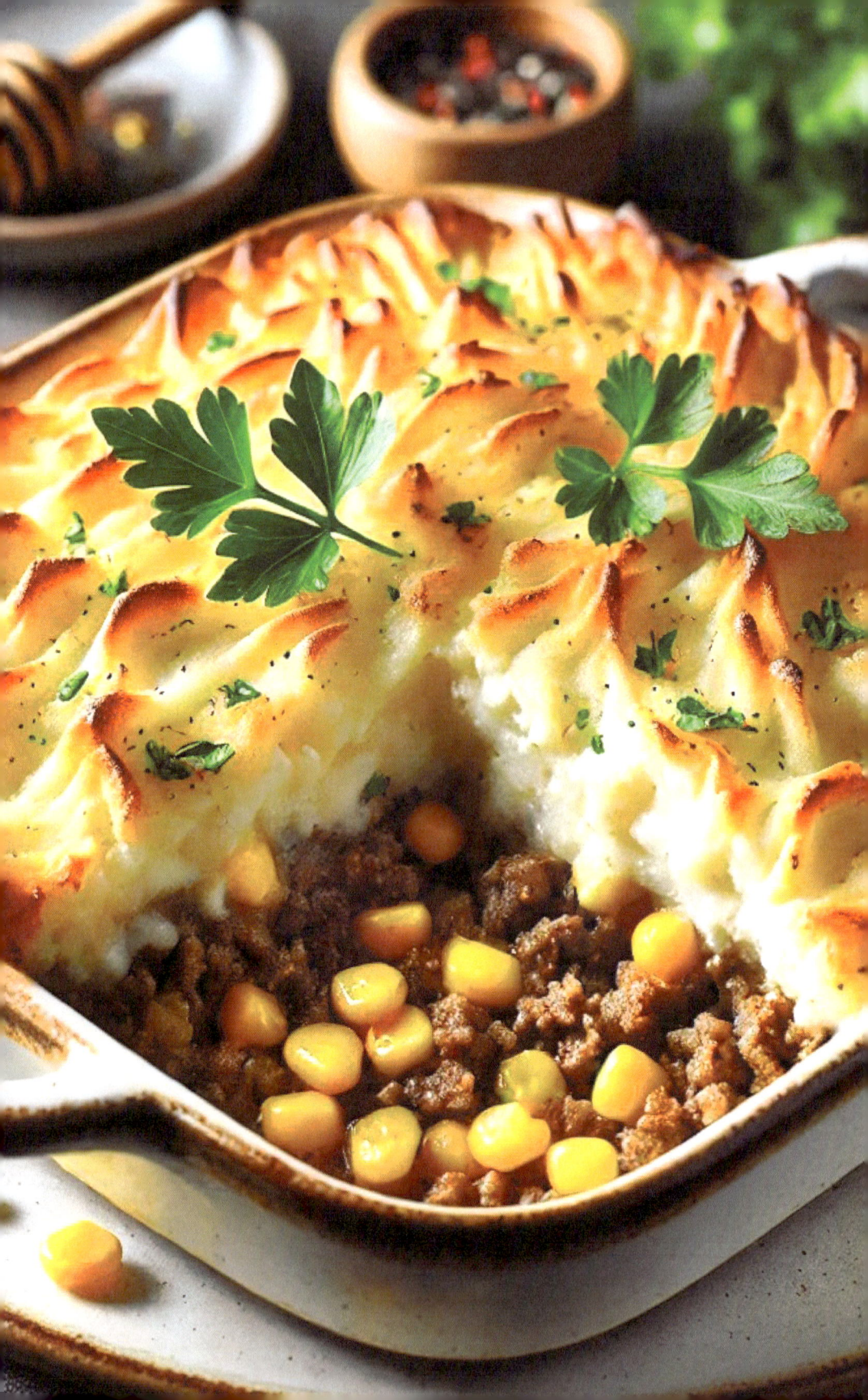

French Canadian Shepherd's Pie

This comforting food is great on a cold day or when you want something hearty to feed a small crowd.

Ingredients:
1 tablespoon olive oil
1 pound lean ground beef (or ground turkey)
1 medium white onion (chopped)
1 teaspoon salt
1 teaspoon black pepper
1 14-ounce can of corn (drained)
5-6 medium potatoes, boiled until soft
½ stick butter
1 cup whole milk

Tools You'll Need:
Large skillet
Large bowl
Potato masher or electric mixer
Measuring cups and spoons
Large baking dish

Step-by-Step Instructions:

1 Preheat oven to 350 degrees and mash potatoes.
Mash potatoes in a large bowl with a potato masher or electric mixer with 1 cup milk and ½ stick of butter.

2 Cook your meat.
Heat oil in a large skillet and sauté onions for 3 to 4 minutes. Add ground beef (or turkey) and cook until brown and cooked through. Add salt and pepper and pour mixture into a baking dish. Pour canned corn on top.

3 Spread mashed potatoes on top and bake for 35 minutes until golden brown.

Tips for Accessibility:
If you don't want to boil potatoes, after scrubbing and drying them pierce them several times with a fork and microwave for 4-5 minutes, flip, and microwave for 4 minutes again until soft.

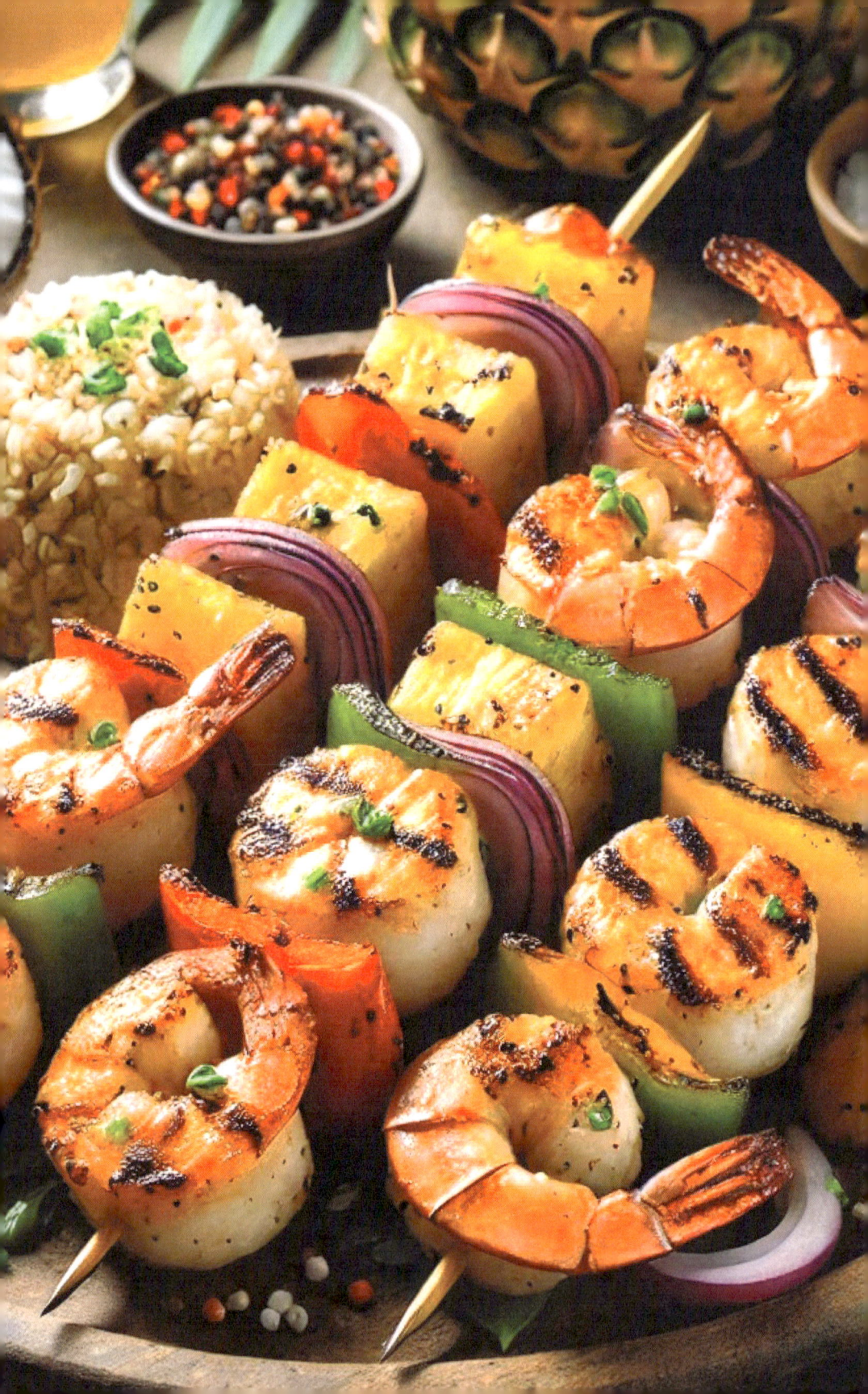

Hawaiian Scallops and Shrimp Kebab

Kebabs are great as appetizers for a party or for a quick, protein-rich meal. If you don't have metal skewers, make sure you soak your wooden skewers so they don't burn on the grill.

Ingredients:
1 pound large shrimp (peeled and de-veined)
½ pound scallops
1 red bell pepper, cut into one inch pieces
1 green bell pepper, cut into one inch pieces
1 small can pineapple (in water), cut into wedges
½ cup rice vinegar
2 teaspoons sesame oil
2 teaspoons powdered ginger
3 tablespoons soy sauce

Tools You'll Need:
Wooden (or metal) skewers (about 6)
Basting brush
Measuring cups and spoons
Medium mixing bowl
Grill (or grill plate for a stovetop)

Step-by-Step Instructions:

1 **Prepare skewers.**
   If using wooden skewers, soak them in warm water for 15 minutes to prevent them from burning during grilling.

2 **Thread your skewers.**
   Thread the shrimp, scallops, peppers, and pineapple on the skewers.

3 **Make the basting sauce.**
   In a medium-sized mixing bowl, combine rice vinegar, sesame oil, ginger, and soy sauce. Mix well.

4 **Prepare your grill.**
   Prepare an outside grill with an oiled rack set 4 inches above the heat source. Place the skewers on the grill and baste with some of the sauce using a brush. Grill kebabs for 5 to 6 minutes, turning and basting regularly with the sauce until warm. Heat remaining basting sauce in the microwave or over a stovetop, and serve with the skewers.

Tips for Accessibility:
Use ready-to-eat shrimp so you don't have to cut or de-vein them.
Have someone help you with the grilling if you aren't comfortable with open flame cooking.

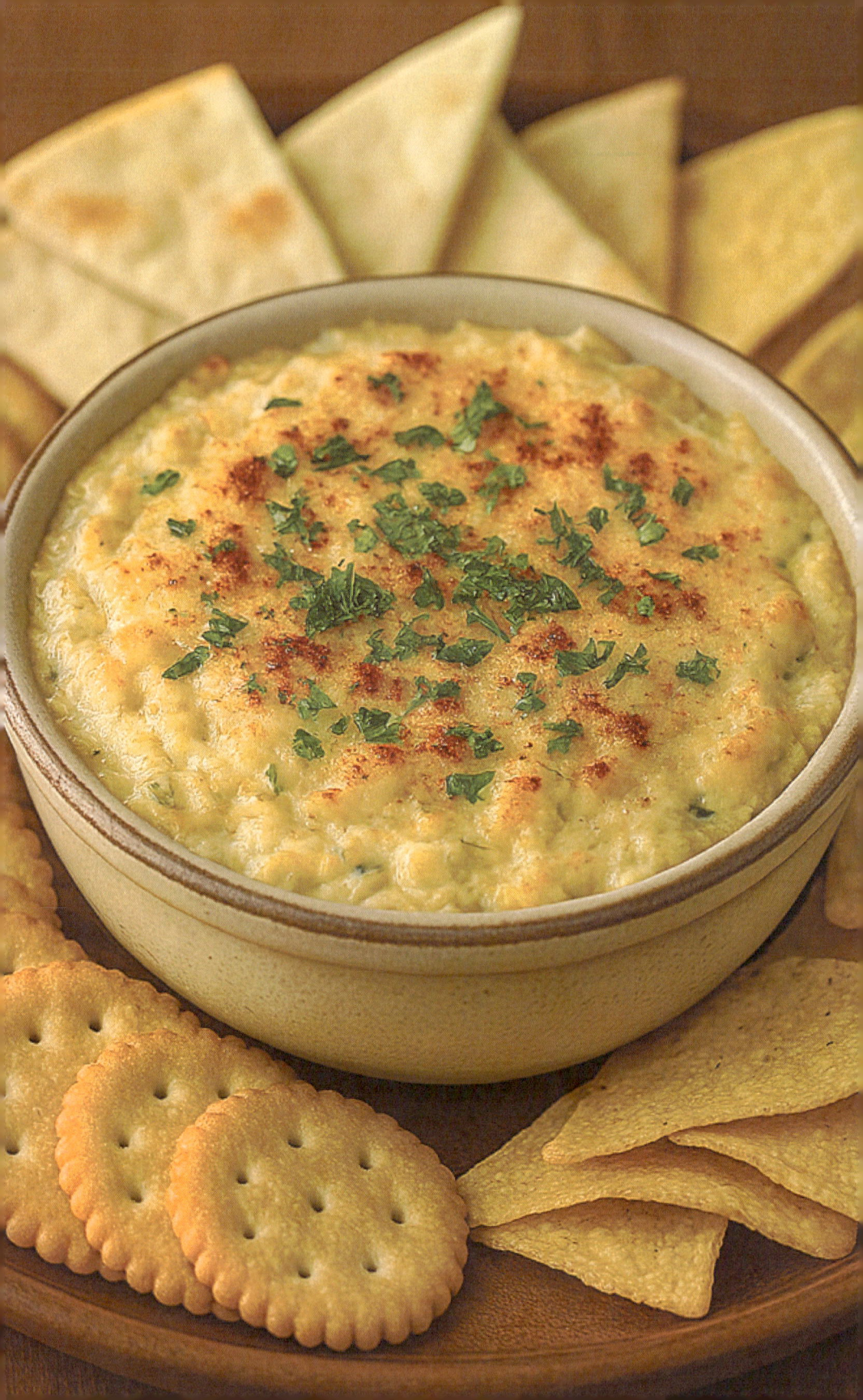

Hot Artichoke Dip

Artichoke dip is an instant crowd-pleaser. Serve it in a small bowl surrounded by your favorite chips, pita bread, or assorted crackers.

Ingredients:

1 8-ounce package of cream cheese, softened
1 cup mayonnaise
1 14-ounce can of artichoke hearts (whole, halves, or quarters), drained and coarsely chopped
¼ cup chopped onion
1 cup grated Parmesan cheese
1 cup grated mozzarella cheese
1 teaspoon garlic salt
1 teaspoon paprika
1 handful chopped parsley (optional) for garnish

Tools You'll Need:

Large bowl
Electric mixer
Small to medium oven-proof dish
4 small cups or bowls

Step-by-Step Instructions:

1 Preheat oven to 350 degrees.

2 Mix your dip ingredients.
In a large bowl, use an electric mixer to beat cream cheese until smooth. Blend in mayonnaise, onion, and chopped artichoke. Mix in Parmesan, mozzarella, and garlic salt and beat at high speed until mixture is smooth. Pour into an oven-safe baking dish.

3 Bake at 350 degrees for 25 to 30 minutes until hot and bubbly.
Garnish with parsley and sprinkle with paprika. Serve with your favorite chips, crackers, tortillas, or pita bread.

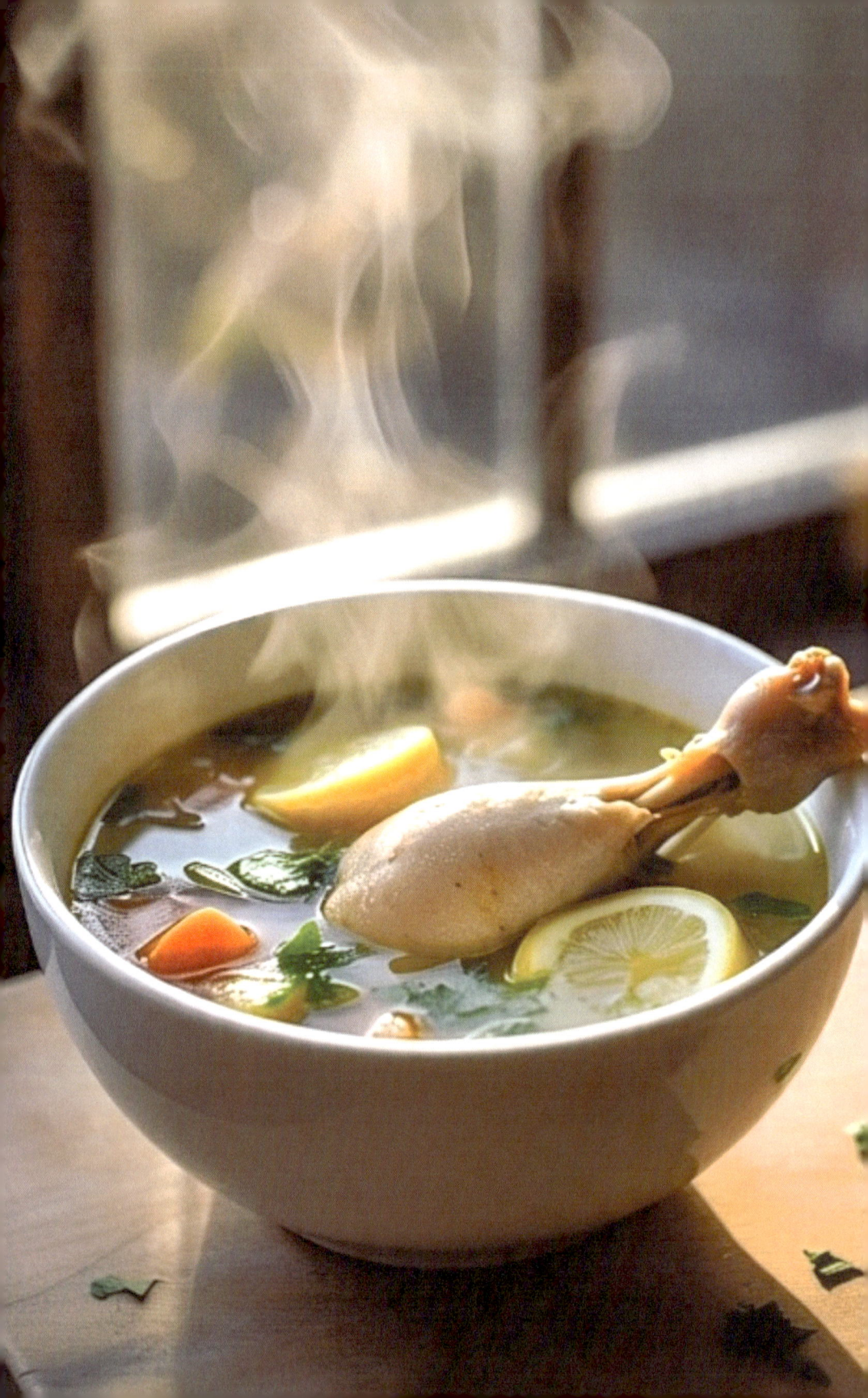

Instant Pot Chicken Soup

There's nothing like a hot bowl of homemade soup on a cold day — or when you have a cold! This one features healthy veggies and fresh chicken, and with an Instant Pot you can have it ready in way less time than cooking it over a stove.

Ingredients:
6 pieces of chicken (boneless, skinless thighs and breasts; about 1 ½ to 2 pounds)
Yukon Gold potatoes, peeled and chopped
½ bag frozen corn
4 cups water
4 cups chicken broth
1 carrot (chopped)
1 piece of celery (chopped)
1 yellow squash (sliced)
½ red tomato, sliced into quarters
¼ onion (chopped)
1 tablespoon olive oil
1 teaspoon chicken bouillon powder
Salt and pepper to taste

Tools You'll Need:
Instant Pot (preferably one with multiple cooking settings)
Spoon
Measuring cups and spoons

Step-by-Step Instructions:

1 Sauté your veggies in the Instant Pot.
Using the sauté feature on your Instant Pot, heat one tablespoon of olive oil and sauté your onion, celery, and carrots until they have softened. Turn off the sautè feature.

2 Prepare ingredients in your Instant Pot.
Place chicken pieces in the pot, along with chicken bouillon powder, 4 cups of chicken broth and 4 cups of water. Add in squash, tomato, frozen corn, and pota-toes. Turn on the "poultry" program, add 20 minutes to the time, and press start. Once it is done cooking, allow the pressure to naturally release before you open the lid. Season to taste with salt and pepper. You can freeze leftovers for up to one month.

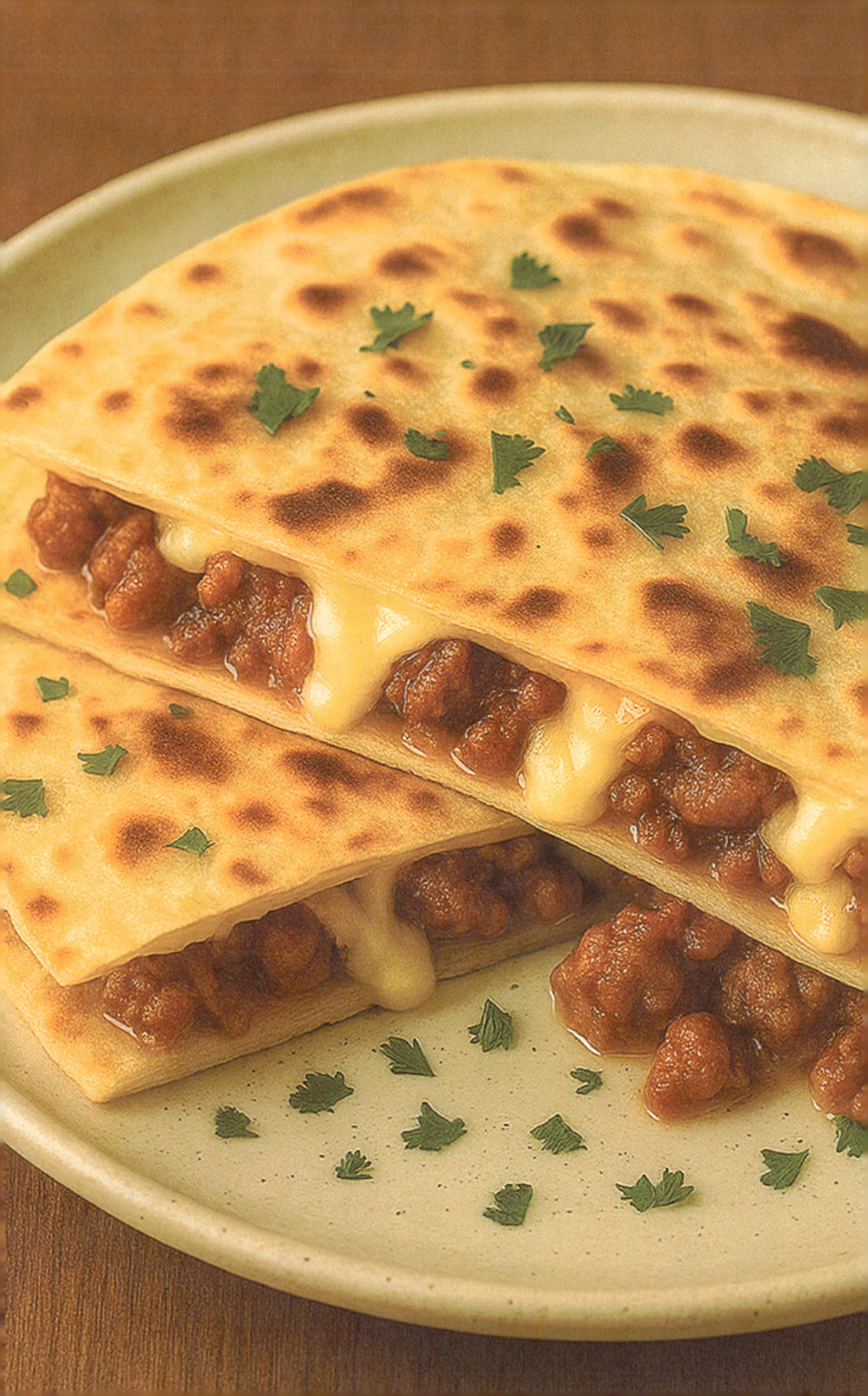

Longaniza Quesadillas

Longaniza, similar to chorizo, is a delicious sausage often used in Latin cuisine. Longaniza has a slightly different seasoning from chorizo, but you can use either for this recipe. If you don't like a lot of heat, look for a package labeled "mild."

Ingredients:
1 package of El Mexicano Longaniza (or similar)
1 ½ cup mozzarella or cheddar cheese (or a mixture of both)
4 flour tortillas
2 teaspoons of water

Tools You'll Need:
Medium skillet
Spoon
Grill pan or large skillet
Measuring cups and spoons
Spatula

Step-by-Step Instructions:

1 Cook your Longaniza.

Heat your medium skillet over medium heat and place the longaniza, breaking it apart with a spoon. Add two tablespoons of water as you cook the sausage. Stir for about 10 minutes until sausage is fully cooked. Turn off heat.

2 Make your quesadillas.

Warm a grill pan or large skillet over low to medium heat. Warm a tortilla on one side, then gently flip onto the other side. Add handful of cheese and a spoonful of Longaniza on one side of the tortilla and allow to warm slightly before using a spatula to fold over the other side of the tortilla. Once the cheese starts to melt, flip the quesadilla and allow to brown on the other side. Repeat this process for each tortilla. You can cut each quesadilla into triangles and top with avocado or salsa if desired.

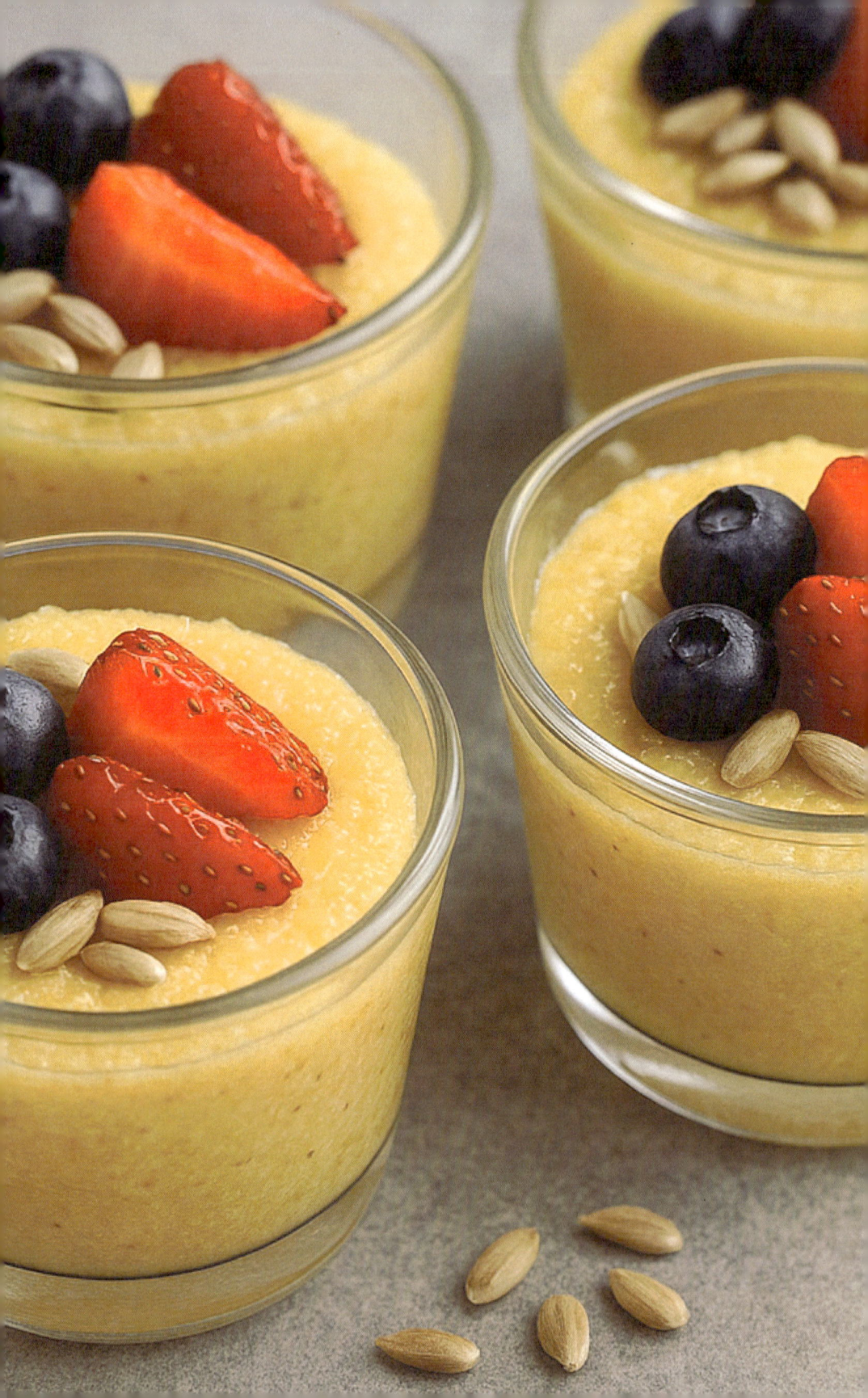

Maple Cornmeal Berry Cups

In Native American cultures, corn is a staple. Ground cornmeal has a versatile consistency that can be both savory and sweet depending on what you add to it. These berry cups are on the sweet side due to the berries and maple syrup. Use whatever berries you have on hand, but blueberries and strawberries work particularly well.

Ingredients:

(Makes 4 small cups)
½ cup fine cornmeal
1 ½ cups water
¼ teaspoon salt
2 tablespoons maple syrup (or honey)
½ teaspoon cinnamon (optional)
½ cup soft berries (fresh or thawed frozen: blueberries, strawberries, or mixed)
1 tablespoon sunflower seeds (optional topping)

Step-by-Step Instructions:

1 Cook the cornmeal base.
In a small pot, mix the cornmeal, water, and salt. Stir over medium heat until it starts to bubble. Reduce heat and stir constantly for about 5 minutes, until thick and smooth (like warm pudding).

2 Add sweetness and spice.
Stir in the maple syrup and cinnamon (if using). Remove from heat.

3 Scoop into cups.
Spoon the warm mixture evenly into 4 small cups or bowls.

4 Top with berries.
Gently press a few soft berries into the top of each cup. Add a few sunflower seeds for crunch if you like.

5 Cool and serve.
Let cool for 5 minutes. Eat warm with a spoon, or chill in the fridge for a cool, pudding-like treat.

Tools You'll Need:

Small saucepan
Spoon for stirring
Measuring cups and spoons
4 small cups or bowls

Tips for Accessibility:

All ingredients are soft—no chopping needed.

Cornmeal cooks fast and thickens quickly—great sensory feedback!

Berries can be added by hand, like a fun decoration step.

Maple syrup is easy to pour and mix.

Optional steps (like seeds or cinnamon) can be skipped if needed.

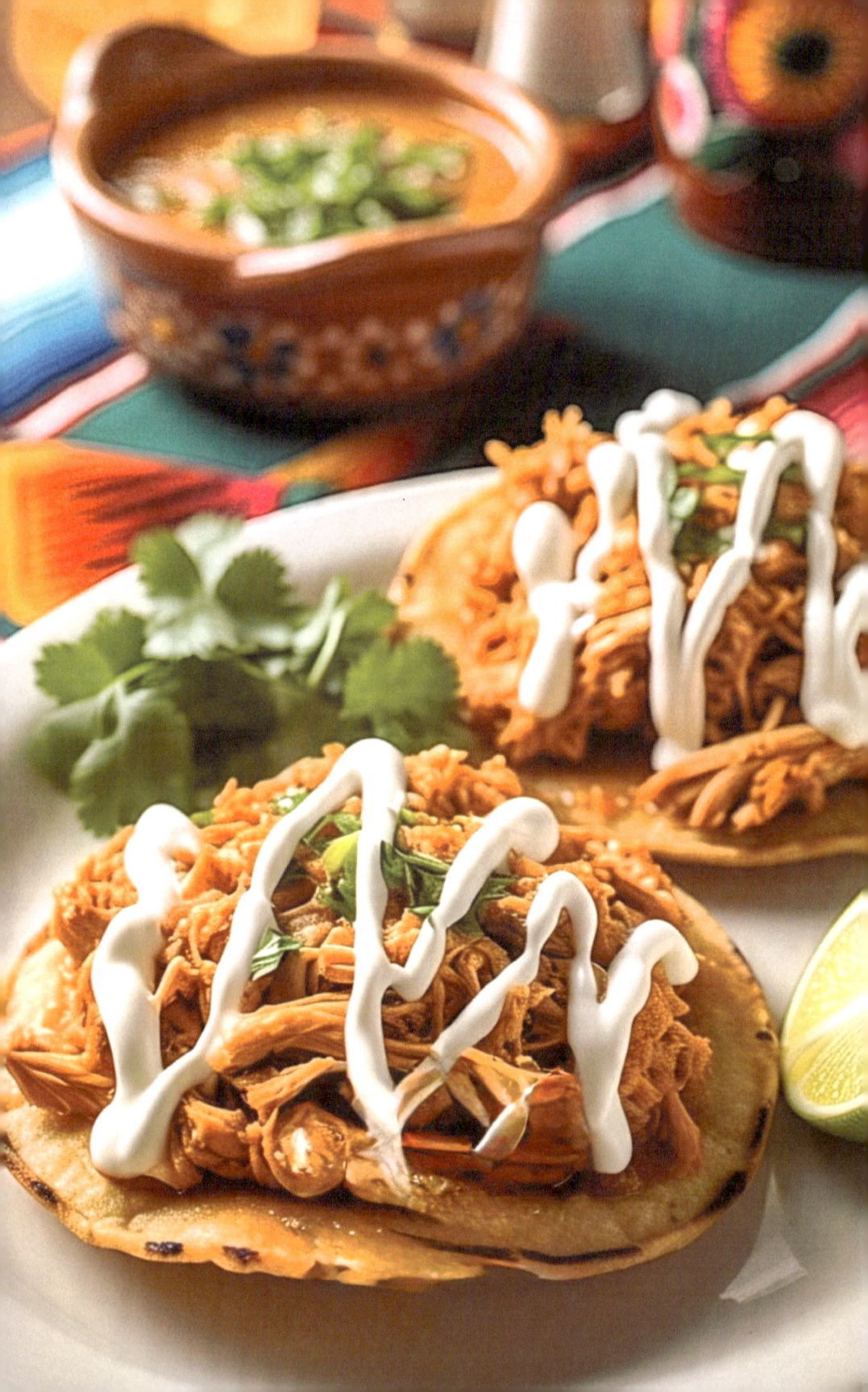

Mexican Tinga

This popular, stew-like Mexican dish hails from Puebla, Mexico, and the vibrant colors and spice from the chipotle and tomato sauce dazzle. If you want to up the heat factor, add some chopped jalapeño peppers to the sauce.

Ingredients:

2 boneless, skinless chicken breasts
1 can chipotle peppers in sauce
2 tomatoes
1 ½ onions
2 garlic cloves (chopped)
Salt to taste
Optional: 1 chopped jalapeño pepper, seeds removed

Tools You'll Need:

Medium pot
Large skillet
Measuring cups and spoons
Slotted spoon
Two forks
Blender

Step-by-Step Instructions:

1 Make your Tinga sauce.

In a medium pot, boil water and then add your chicken breasts, tomatoes, and one onion, along with a large pinch of salt. Once the tomatoes and onion are soft, use a slotted spoon to transfer them to a blender. Reserve one cup of water for the sauce, but continue boiling the chicken until done. Add your can of chipotle peppers and garlic to the blender (and jalapeño if using), along with the cup of reserved water. Blend until desired consistency, adding water if needed. You want the sauce to be thick but not overly chunky.

2 Finish your chicken and combine with Tinga sauce.

Once your chicken is done, remove it with a slotted spoon and place on a cutting board to shred with two forks. Cut the remaining half onion into strips, and place in a large skillet heated with oil over medium heat. Cook until transparent, stirring frequently. Add chicken and Tinga sauce to the skillet and stir until just combined. Cover and let mixture simmer over medium heat for 15 minutes. Serve with tortilla chips, tostadas, or top with avocado.

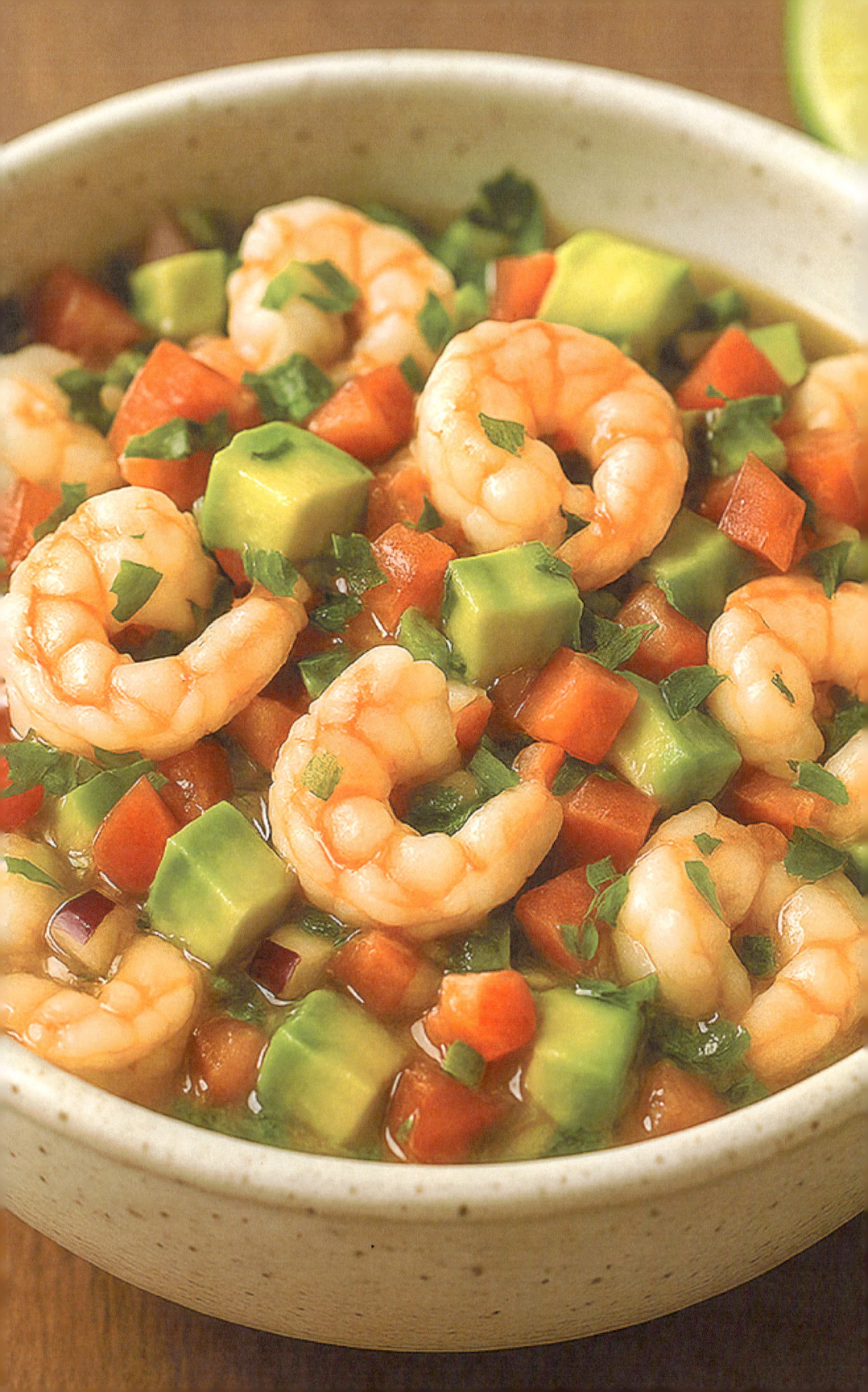

Mexican Shrimp Ceviche

A mild but zesty, no-cook way to enjoy some protein. You can adjust the seasonings to your liking and even add in some red pepper flakes or chopped jalapeño for some heat.

Ingredients:
1 lb. Shrimp (medium to large size)
1 small onion
2 small tomatoes
1 bunch of cilantro
The juice of 3 lemons
Salt and Pepper to taste
Optional: ½ cup diced fresh jalapeño or ½ teaspoon red pepper flakes.

Tools You'll Need:
Medium-sized bowl
Spoon
Measuring cups and spoons
Knife
Cutting Board
Kitchen shears
Colander to wash shrimp thoroughly

Step-by-Step Instructions:

1 **Wash and peel shrimp**
Wash the shrimp thoroughly under cold running water and carefully use your kitchen shears to cut the outer shell lengthwise, stopping when you get to the tail. Peel back the shell from either side of the cut and discard the shell.

2 **Chop your vegetables.**
Chop the cilantro finely and dice the onion. Cut the cucumber and tomato in half lengthwise, then use a spoon to scoop out the seeds in both so the ceviche does not become watery. Dice the remaining cucumber and tomato.

3 **Assemble ceviche.**
In a medium-sized bowl, assemble all ingredients and toss with lemon juice and desired salt and pepper. Enjoy!

Tips for Accessibility:
Use pre-peeled shrimp (you can find them in the frozen foods aisle) if you don't want to peel them.

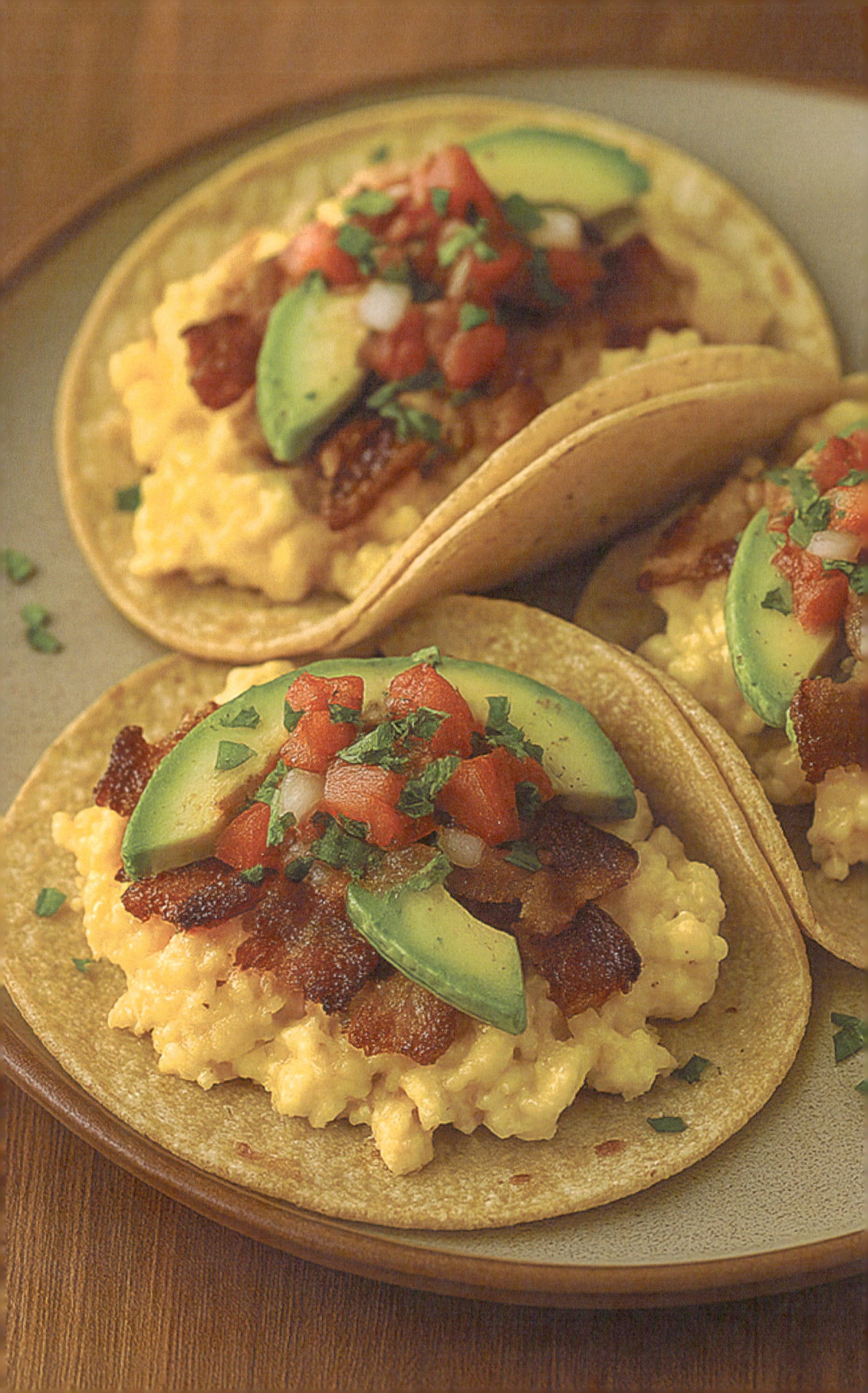

San Diego Sunrise Tacos

Soft breakfast tacos with eggs, avocado, and salsa—fresh and beachy, just like San Diego mornings!

Ingredients:
(Makes 2 tacos)
2 small soft tortillas (corn or flour)
2 eggs
1 small avocado (or use pre-sliced)
2 tablespoons shredded cheese
2 tablespoons mild salsa
1 teaspoon oil or butter
A pinch of salt

Optional Add-ins:
A sprinkle of chopped cilantro
A spoonful of plain yogurt or sour cream
Squeeze of lime

Tools You'll Need:
Frying pan
Spatula
Small bowl and fork
Plate

Tips for Accessibility:
Use pre-cracked eggs or pour from a cup.

Avocado can be sliced with a plastic knife or mashed with a fork.

Use mild salsa with no chunks for easy scooping.

Step-by-Step Instructions:

1 **Scramble the eggs.**
Crack eggs into a bowl and mix with a fork.
Heat a little oil or butter in the pan on medium. Pour in the eggs and stir with a spatula until scrambled and cooked. Turn off heat.

2 **Warm the tortillas**
Place tortillas in the warm pan for 10 seconds on each side or microwave them for 15 seconds to make them soft.

3 **Build the tacos.**
Place warm tortillas on a plate. Add scrambled eggs, sprinkle with cheese, and top with sliced or mashed avocado. Spoon salsa over the top.

4 **Fold and eat.**
Fold each taco gently in half and enjoy warm. Use your hands or a fork—your choice!

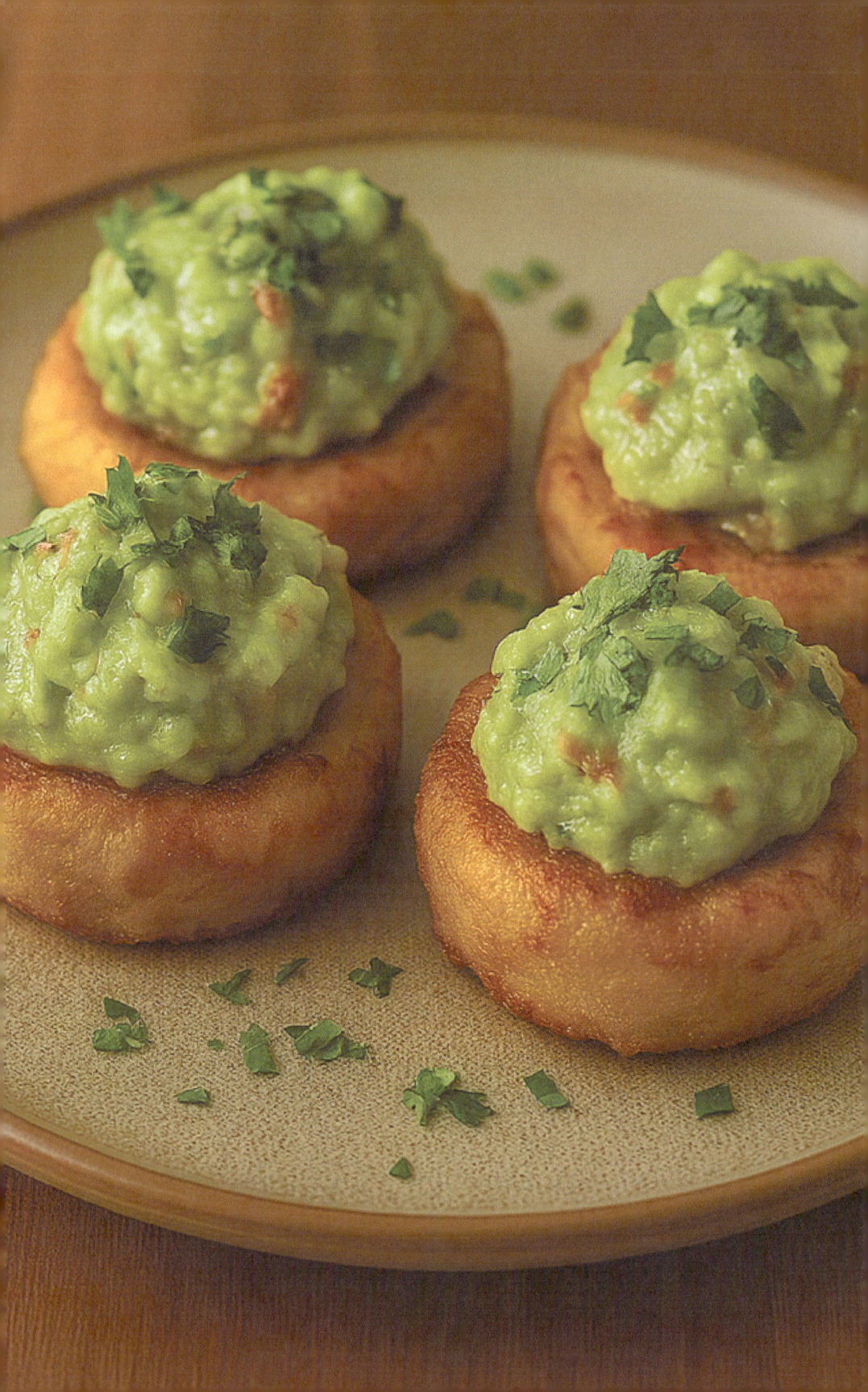

Soft Plantain Mash Bites

A bite-sized version of Dominican mangú, served in small scoops with a hint of garlic and onion—no frying, no knives, and easy to enjoy. This dish is typically served alongside a breakfast meat and some eggs as part of a traditional Dominican breakfast.

Ingredients:
(Makes 6–8 bites)

1 large ripe plantain (yellow with a few brown spots)
1 tablespoon butter or oil
1 tablespoon onion flakes or 1 tablespoon pre-cooked onion
¼ teaspoon garlic powder
A pinch of salt
Optional: 1 tablespoon sour cream or plain yogurt (for dipping)

Tools You'll Need:
Microwave-safe bowl or small pot
Spoon
Fork or potato masher
Small plate or tray

Step-by-Step Instructions:

1 Cook the Plantain
Peel the ripe plantain (ask for help if needed) and slice into chunks.

Microwave Method: Place in a bowl with 2 tablespoons water, cover loosely, and microwave for 4–5 minutes until very soft.

Stovetop Method: Boil in water for 10–12 minutes until fork-tender.

2 Mash the Mixture
Drain any extra water. Add butter, onion flakes, garlic powder, and a pinch of salt. Mash with a fork or masher until smooth and creamy.

3 Shape into Bites
Let the plantain mash cool slightly. Scoop small spoonfuls onto a plate or tray. You can shape them into little patties or leave them as soft dollops.

4 Serve and Dip
Serve warm or room temp with a little yogurt or sour cream for dipping.

Tips for Accessibility:
Ripe plantains are soft and easy to mash.

Microwave cooking avoids frying and boiling water.

No knives needed—just spooning and mashing.

Easy to shape and serve by hand.

Great sensory feedback: warm, creamy, and lightly sweet-savory.

41

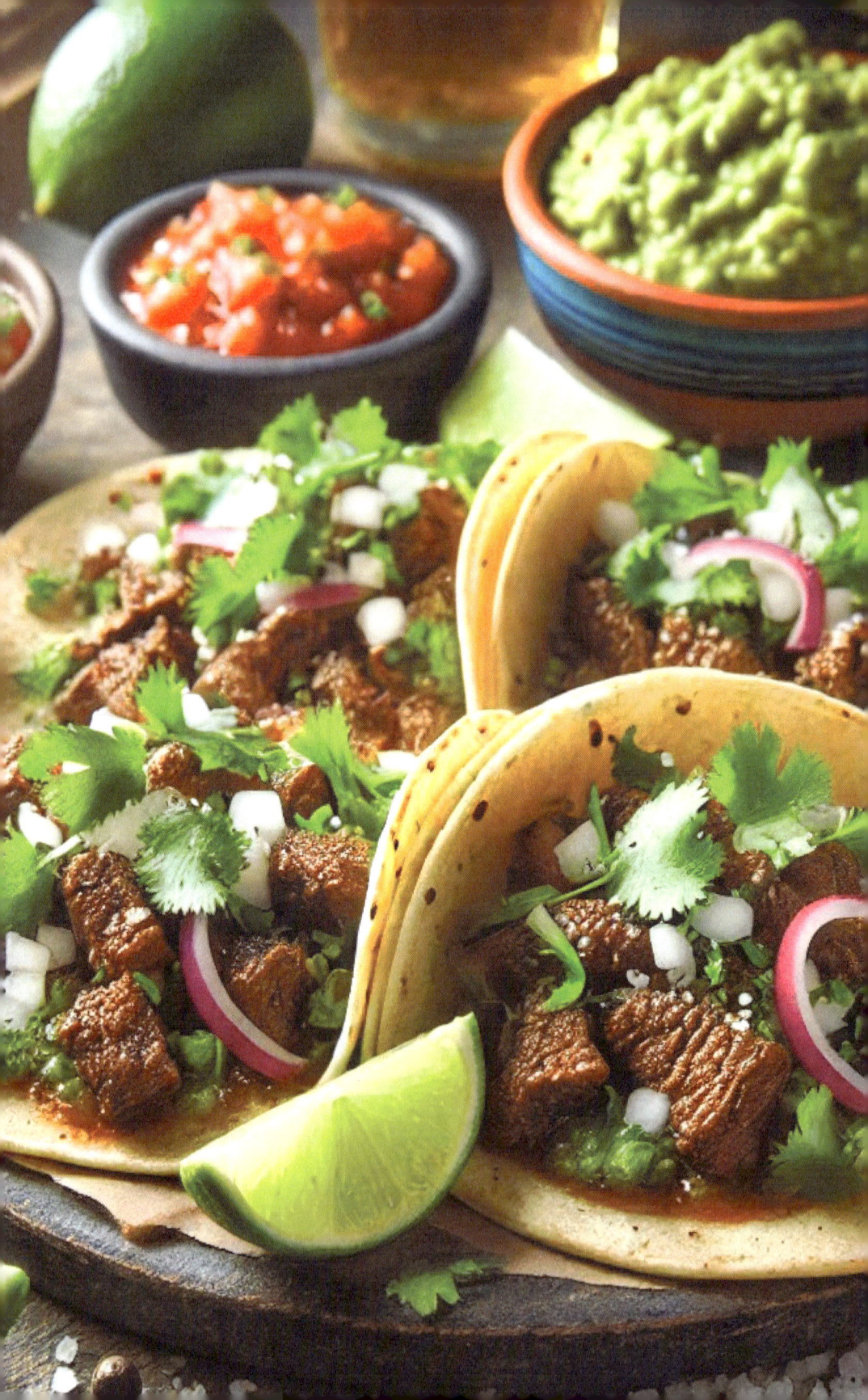

Tuesday Beef Street Tacos

If you haven't designated Tuesday as "Tuesday Taco Day," now is the time. These tasty tacos come together super quickly, and you can pile them high with whatever toppings you have on hand: avocado, shredded cheese, lettuce, tomato, jalapeño, and more.

Ingredients:

1 pound of ground beef
1 package taco seasoning (I recommend Mc-Cormick or Old El Paso)
1 small onion (chopped)
2 garlic cloves (chopped)
1 teaspoon oil
4 cups chicken broth
1 teaspoon tomato paste
6-8 corn tortillas

Tools You'll Need:

Medium skillet
Spoon
Measuring cups and spoons
Small bowl
Grill pan or small pan

Step-by-Step Instructions:

1 Cook your beef.

Heat one teaspoon oil over medium heat. Add chopped onion and sauté until soft, then add garlic and sauté until fragrant. Add beef and cook, breaking apart with a spoon for 4 to 5 minutes.

2 Add taco seasoning and tomato paste.

In a small bowl, add a teaspoon of tomato paste to 1 to 2 tablespoons of warm water and dissolve, then add to the meat mixture along with your taco seasoning. Continue cooking, stirring regularly, until meat is cooked all the way through.

3 Warm tortillas and serve.

Spray some Pam or other oil on a grill pan or small pan and warm up your corn tortillas until lightly browned on either side. Prepare your toppings and add them to your tacos. Enjoy!

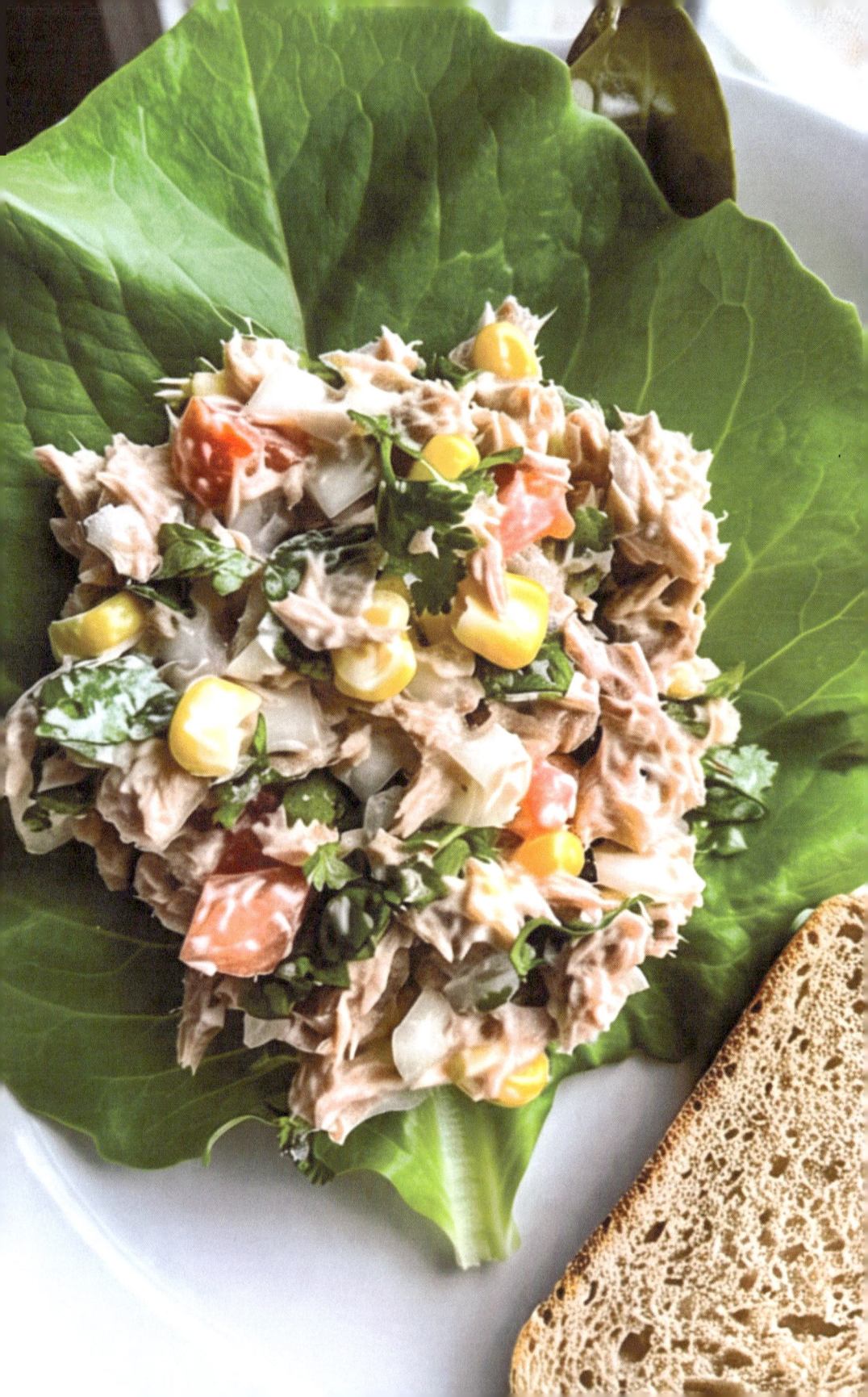

Tuna Salad

It's always good to have a good tuna salad recipe on hand for sandwiches, salads, or for days when you just don't know what to eat for lunch. I like to put whatever vegetables I have in the fridge in mine, but celery, corn, and red onion are particularly tasty options. If you happen to have any fresh herbs like dill or parsley on hand, chop them up and add them for extra flavor.

Ingredients:
2 small cans of tuna (in water)
1 cinnamon stick
1 can of mixed vegetables
1 can of corn
2 tablespoons mayonnaise
Salt and pepper to taste
Optional: ¼ cup chopped fresh herbs

Tools You'll Need:
Medium bowl
Measuring cups and spoons
Spatula or wooden spoon

Step-by-Step Instructions:

1 **Drain your tuna fish.**
Open your tuna cans and drain the water from each one.

2 **Assemble your tuna salad.**
In a medium bowl, mix together tuna, vegetables, herbs if using, and mayonnaise. Season with salt and pepper to taste. Serve with chips, make a sandwich, or put a spoonful on salad.

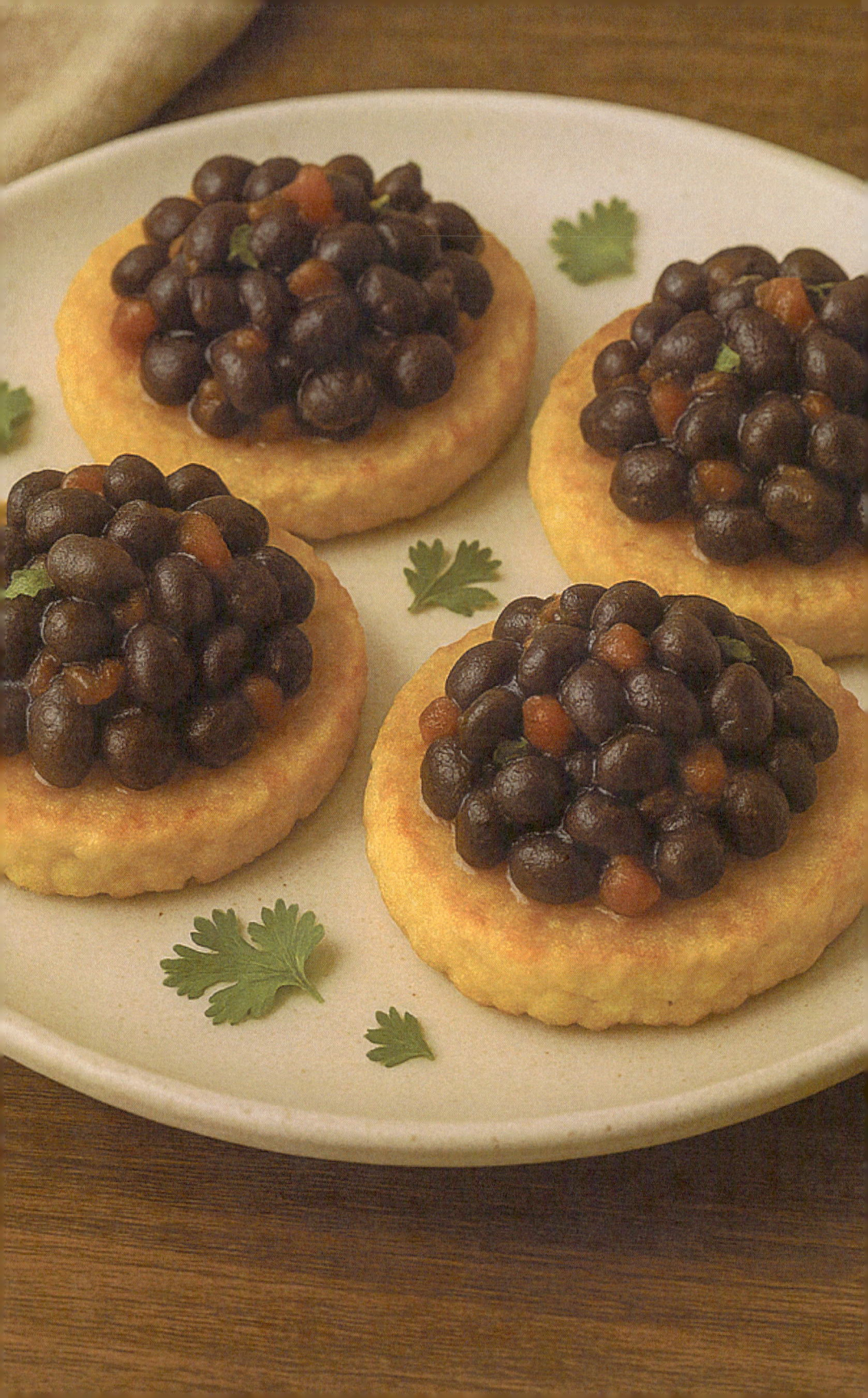

Mini Panama Corn Cakes with Bean Topping

Soft, golden corn patties topped with seasoned beans and a touch of lime—like a tropical tostada, made easy!

Ingredients:
(Makes 6 mini cakes)

For the corn cakes:
1 cup instant cornmeal (like PAN or masa harina)
¾ cup warm water
A pinch of salt
1 tablespoon oil or butter (for brushing)

For the topping:
½ cup canned black beans (drained and rinsed)
2 tablespoons corn (frozen or canned)
1 tablespoon plain yogurt or sour cream
1 teaspoon lime juice (optional)
A pinch of garlic powder and salt

Tools You'll Need:
Bowl and spoon
Baking tray or non-stick pan
Fork (for mashing beans)

Tips for Accessibility:
Cornmeal dough is fun and safe to handle—like play-dough!

No sharp tools or stovetop frying required.

Bean topping can be mashed with a fork and mixed in one bowl.

Small portions are easy to plate, share, and eat with hands or a spoon.

Step-by-Step Instructions:

1 Make the corn dough.
In a bowl, mix the cornmeal, warm water, and salt. Stir until it feels like soft playdough. Let it rest for 2 minutes.

2 Shape the cakes.
Divide into 6 small balls. Flatten each into a patty, about the size of a cookie.

3 Bake or pan-toast.
Lightly brush the tops with oil or butter.

Bake at 180°C (350°F) on a tray for 12–15 minutes, flipping once.

Or cook on a dry pan over medium heat for 3–4 minutes per side, until lightly golden.

4 Make the bean topping.
In a bowl, mash the beans slightly with a fork. Mix in corn, yogurt, garlic powder, lime juice, and a pinch of salt.

5 Assemble your cakes.
Once corn cakes are cool enough to touch, add a spoonful of bean topping to each one. Serve on a plate!

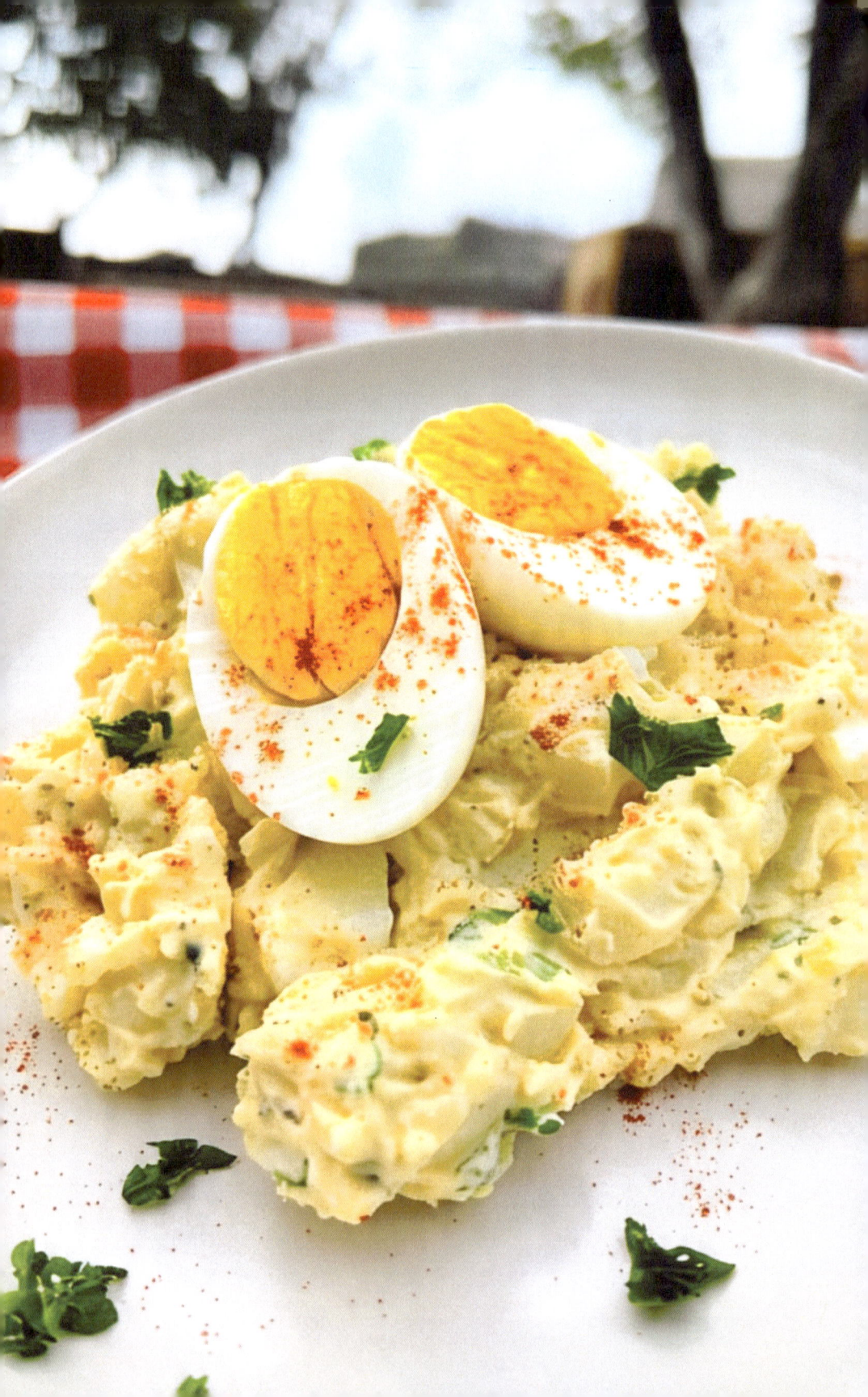

Potato Egg Salad

This BBQ staple is a hit for a reason. The creaminess from the cheese and the egg yolks pairs perfectly with potatoes. When you boil your eggs, make sure to make more than the recipe calls for so you can have some one hand for a snack.

Ingredients:

4 medium-sized Yukon gold or Russet potatoes
5 eggs
3 tablespoons light mayonnaise
2 tablespoons of Parmesan cheese or Cotija shredded cheese
1 teaspoon garlic powder
Salt and pepper to taste

Tools You'll Need:

Medium pots
Measuring cups and spoons
Spatula or wooden spoon
Slotted spoon
Large bowl
Medium bowl (filled with ice and water)

Step-by-Step Instructions:

1 Hard-boil your eggs.
   In a medium pot, fill the water so it covers your eggs by one inch. Bring to a boil, then turn off the heat, cover, and let stand for 10 minutes. Using a slotted spoon, remove your eggs and place them in the ice bath in the medium bowl until cool, then peel and set aside.

2 Boil your potatoes.
   Dump out the water from the eggs. Then fill the pot again with enough water so that the potatoes have one inch of water covering them. Add a large pinch of salt to the water and bring to a boil. Reduce heat to a simmer and keep covered until potatoes are fork tender, roughly 15 minutes. Remove potatoes with a slotted spoon and rub off skin with a paper towel, then chop into bite-sized pieces.

3 Assemble your potato salad.
   In a large bowl, gently mash your eggs using a fork or spoon. Add the potatoes, garlic powder, mayonnaise, and cheese and mix. Season to taste with salt and pepper.

Slow Cooker Chicken Tacos

These pulled chicken tacos are zesty, flavorful, and can easily be made ahead of time for a dinner party or meal prep. Add spice according to your taste, and use whatever toppings you have on hand. Try putting all the toppings in small bowls side by side on a counter to create your own taco bar.

Ingredients:

2 pounds boneless, skinless chicken thighs
1 small onion (chopped)
2 jalapeño pepper (chopped)
2 garlic cloves (chopped)
½ cup chicken broth
1 tablespoon olive oil
1 teaspoon oregano
1 teaspoon cayenne pepper (or more if you like it spicy!)
½ teaspoon cumin
1 teaspoon paprika
1 teaspoon salt
1 teaspoon black pepper
Corn tortillas (warmed) for serving

Tools You'll Need:

Crockpot
Small frying pan
Wooden spoon
Small bowl
Slotted spoon
Cutting board
Measuring cups and spoons

Step-by-Step Instructions:

1 **Put chicken in crockpot with spices.**
   Place chicken thighs in a crockpot. In a small bowl, mix the oregano, cayenne, cumin, paprika, salt, and pepper. Rub the chicken evenly with the spice mixture.

2 **Cook your vegetables.**
   Place oil in a small frying pan and heat over medium-high heat. Add onion and jalapeño pepper. Cook for a few minutes, stirring regularly, and add more oil if the veggies start to burn. Add garlic and cook another minute, stirring often. Add this mixture to the crockpot. Add the chicken broth to the hot pan and scrape up the browned bits from the bottom. Pour the mixture directly into the crockpot.

3 **Cook on low for 4 to 5 hours.**
   Cook your chicken until the chicken breaks apart easily with a fork. Remove your chicken with a slotted spoon and use a fork to shred it, then place it in a bowl or return it to the crockpot to serve.

4 Assemble your taco bar.

Place chicken, fresh diced onions, diced bell pepper, shredded cheese, cilantro, and salsa into separate bowls. Place a plate of warmed tortillas next to the bowls and assemble your tacos as desired. You can also just freeze or refrigerate your pulled chicken until ready to heat and eat.

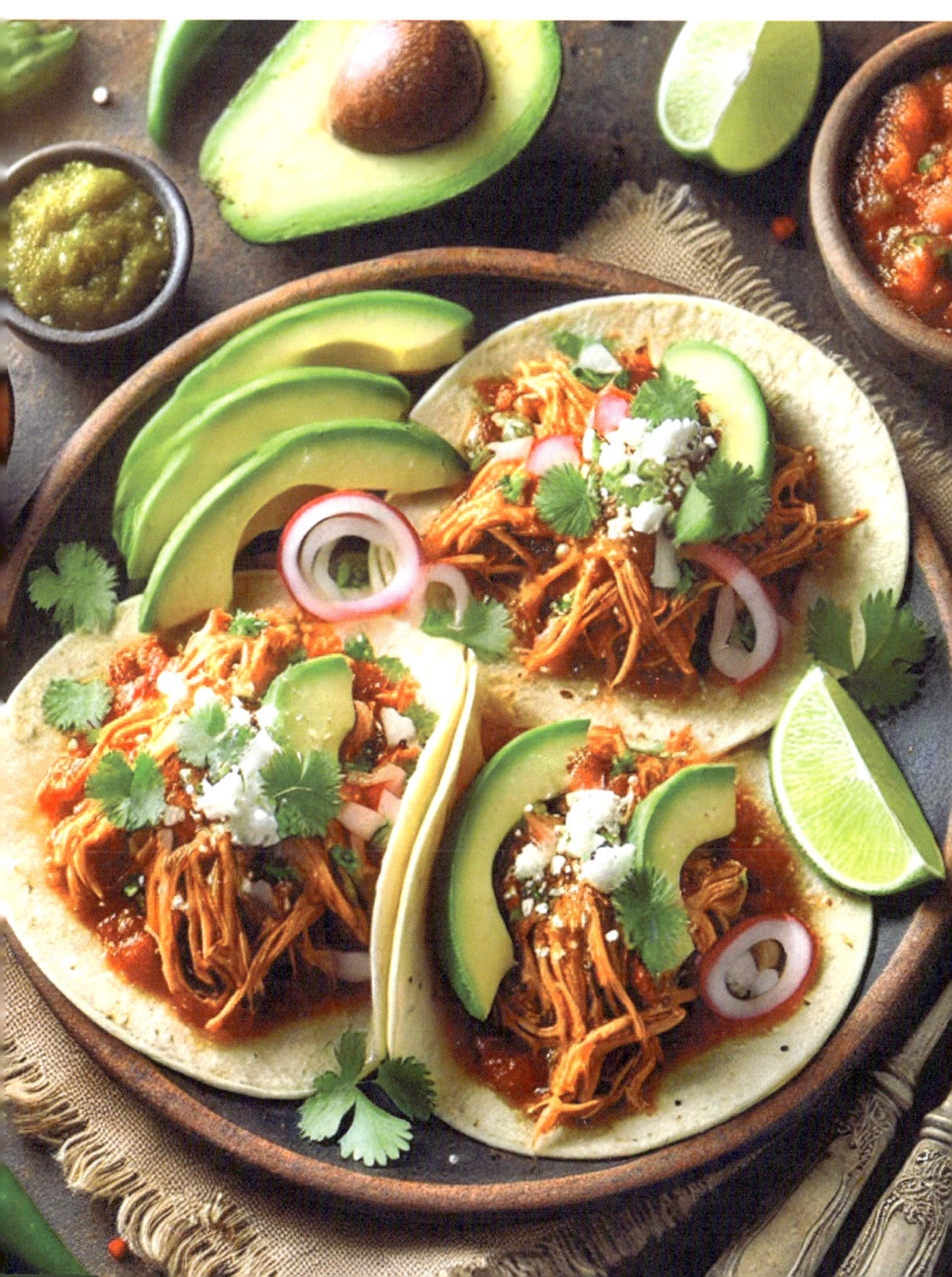

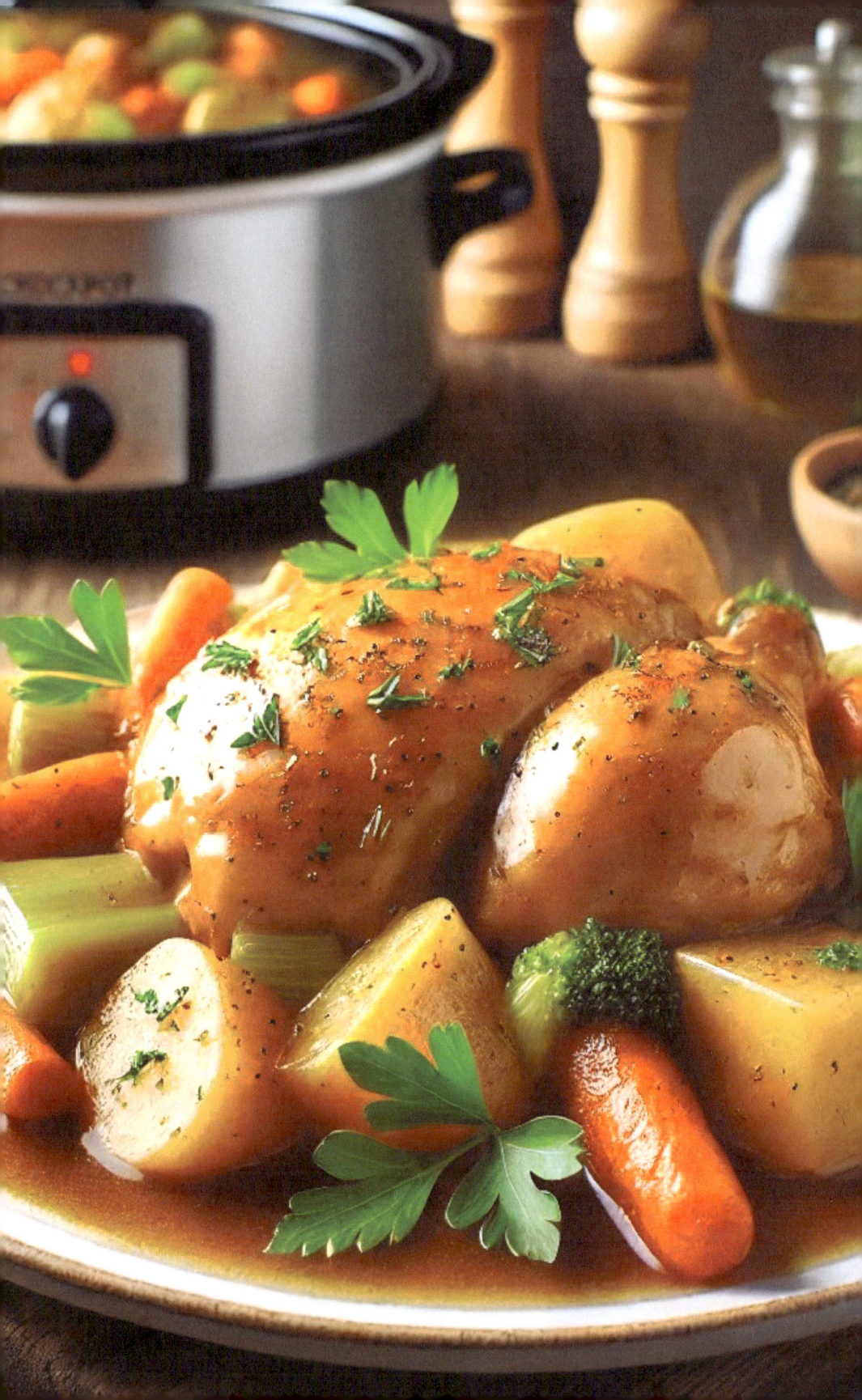

Spenser's American Homestyle Crockpot Chicken

I love to make this recipe for my family and friends. It's hearty, delicious, and full of American comfort food goodness. If you aren't comfortable cutting a whole chicken, either ask a butcher to do it for you or use two pounds of boneless, skinless chicken breasts instead of a whole chicken.

Ingredients:
1 whole chicken, cleaned and cut apart. (or 2 pounds boneless chicken breasts)
1 can of cream of chicken soup
1 cup water
4 russet or Yukon gold potatoes, washed, peeled and chopped into cubes
2 cups baby carrots
½ cup chopped onion
1 tablespoon black pepper
½ tablespoon salt
1 tablespoon garlic powder

Tools You'll Need:
Crockpot
Spoon
Measuring cups and spoons
Small bowl

Tips for Accessibility:
Use chicken breasts instead of a whole chicken to avoid cutting.

Step-by-Step Instructions:

1 Prepare your chicken for the crockpot.
Sprinkle your chicken liberally with garlic powder and black pepper and place it in the crockpot.

2 Place the rest of your ingredients in the crockpot.
In a small bowl, mix one cup of water with your cream of chicken soup, and pour over the chicken. Add in carrots, onion, and potatoes. Sprinkle with salt and stir.

3 Cook on low for 6 hours.
Ladle onto plates and serve with salad and some crusty bread.

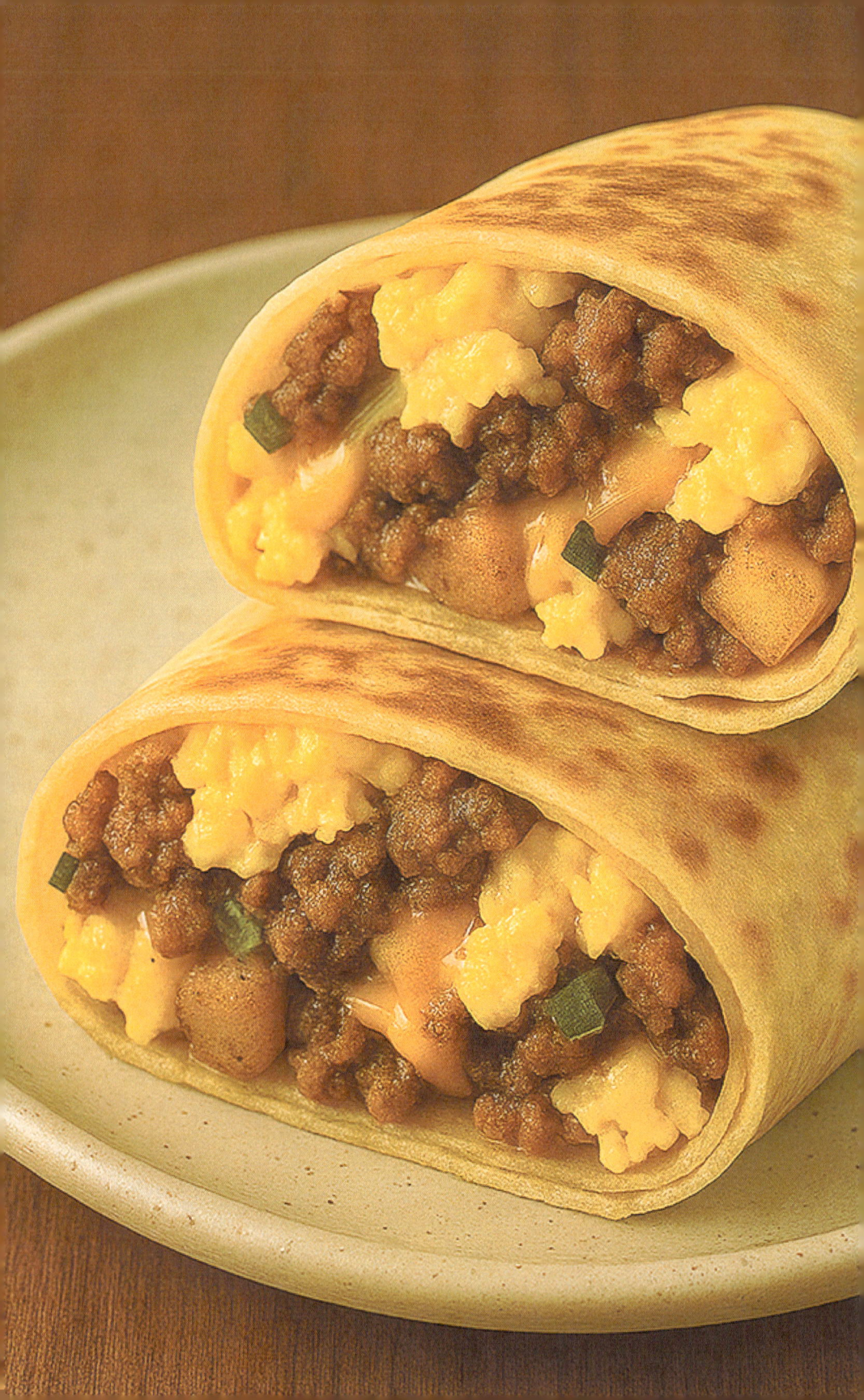

Ultimate Breakfast Burrito

Breakfast burritos are super filling, and surprisingly easy to make. I like to use Longaniza, turkey bacon, and eggs in mine. Fill yours with whatever you like: sausage, home fries, salsa, eggs; just make sure you have a sturdy enough flour tortilla to hold it all!

Ingredients:
1 whole chicken, cleaned and cut apart. (or 2 pounds boneless chicken breasts)
1 can of cream of chicken soup
1 cup water
4 russet or Yukon gold potatoes, washed, peeled and chopped into cubes
2 cups baby carrots
½ cup chopped onion
1 tablespoon black pepper
½ tablespoon salt
1 tablespoon garlic powder

Tools You'll Need:
Crockpot
Spoon
Measuring cups and spoons
Small bowl

Tips for Accessibility:
Use chicken breasts instead of a whole chicken to avoid cutting.

Step-by-Step Instructions:

1 Prepare your chicken for the crockpot.
   Sprinkle your chicken liberally with garlic powder and black pepper and place it in the crockpot.

2 Place the rest of your ingredients in the crockpot.
   In a small bowl, mix one cup of water with your cream of chicken soup, and pour over the chicken. Add in carrots, onion, and potatoes. Sprinkle with salt and stir.

3 Cook on low for 6 hours.
   Ladle onto plates and serve with salad and some crusty bread.

Europe, Africa & the Middle East

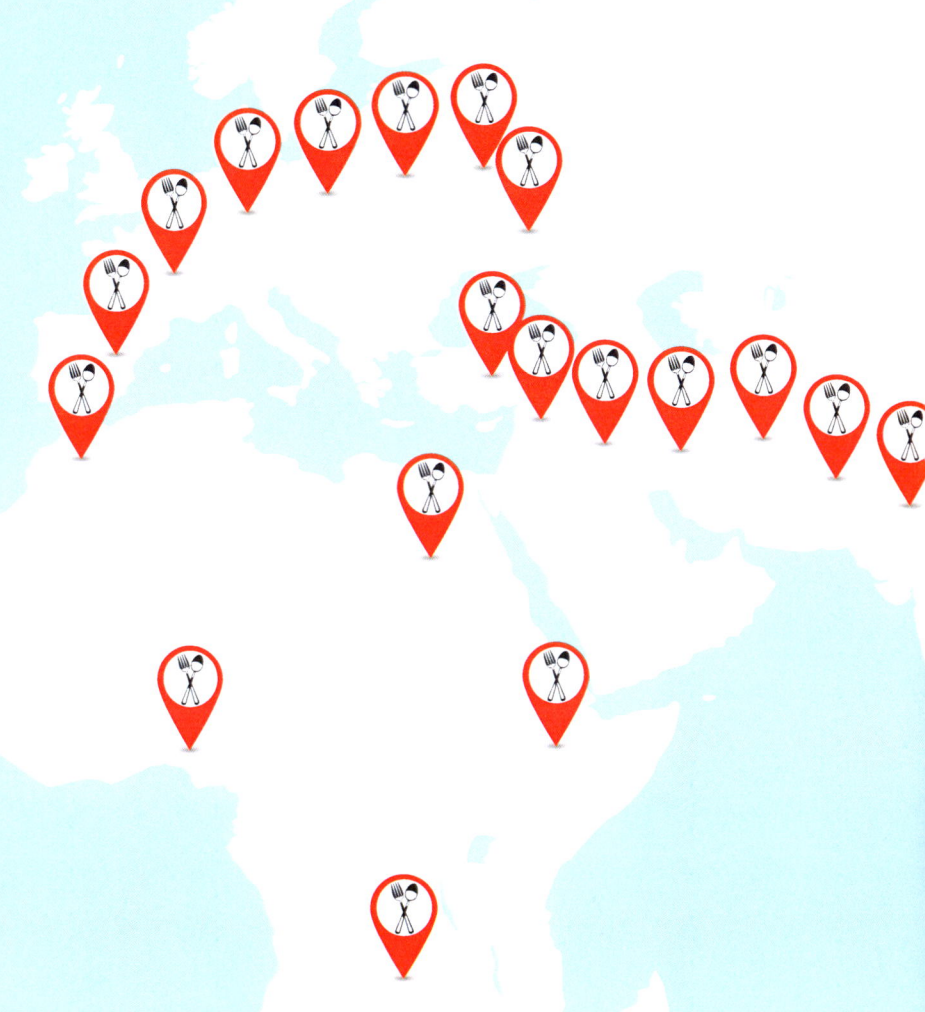

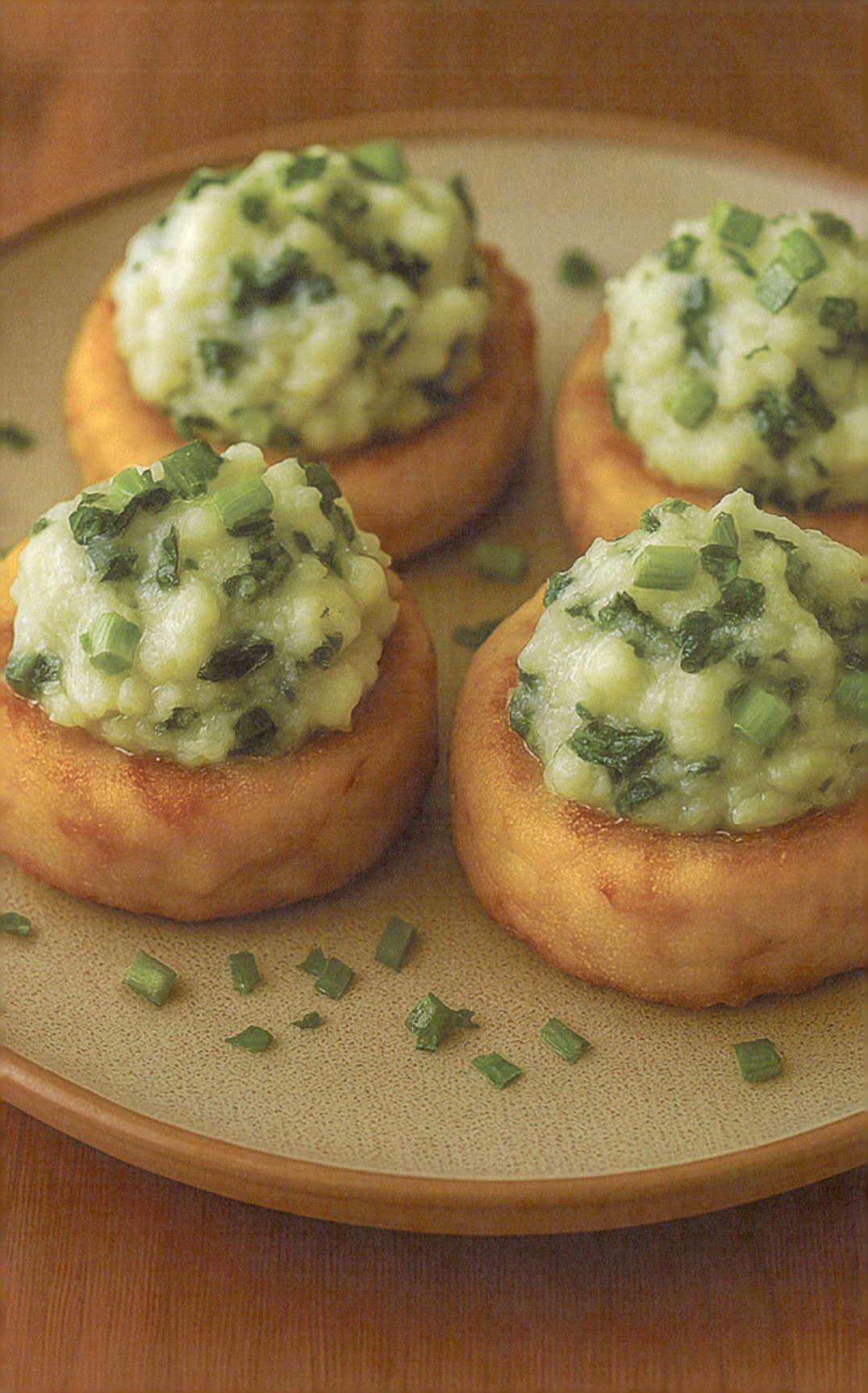

Colcannon Cottage Cups

A cozy Irish mash of potatoes and cabbage, baked into muffin cups with melted cheese on top. Easy to scoop and fun to eat!

Ingredients:
(Makes 6 small cups)
2 medium potatoes (or 2 cups instant mashed potatoes)
1 cup chopped cabbage or kale (fresh or frozen)
¼ cup milk
2 tablespoons butter or margarine
½ cup shredded cheese (cheddar is great!)
Salt and pepper to taste
Optional: ½ cup cooked ground beef or crumbled sausage

Tools You'll Need:
Pot (for boiling or making mashed potatoes)
Spoon
Muffin tin or small oven-safe cups
Oven or toaster oven
Measuring cups and spoons

Tips for Accessibility:
Use instant mashed potatoes for speed and ease.

Pre-cut frozen cabbage works well.

Muffin tins create single portions—no slicing needed!

All ingredients are soft and can be mixed with a spoon.

Safe, feel-good sensory experience—warm, creamy, and cheesy.

Step-by-Step Instructions:

1 **Cook the potatoes.**
Peel and chop the potatoes (ask for help if needed). Boil in water until soft, about 15 minutes. Or use instant mashed potatoes and skip to step 3.

2 **Cook the cabbage.**
While potatoes are boiling, cook cabbage or kale in a little water or steam it until soft (about 5–7 minutes). Drain any extra water.

3 **Mash everything together.**
Drain the cooked potatoes and mash them with butter and milk until smooth. Stir in the cabbage. Add a little salt and pepper.

4 **Fill the cups.**
Preheat oven to 180°C (350°F). Grease a muffin tin or use silicone liners. Spoon the potato mixture into each cup. Press gently to flatten. Add a sprinkle of cheese on top.

5 **Bake and serve.**
Bake for 10–12 minutes until the cheese is melted and golden. Let cool for a few minutes before eating. Serve with a spoon or eat with hands if firm enough!

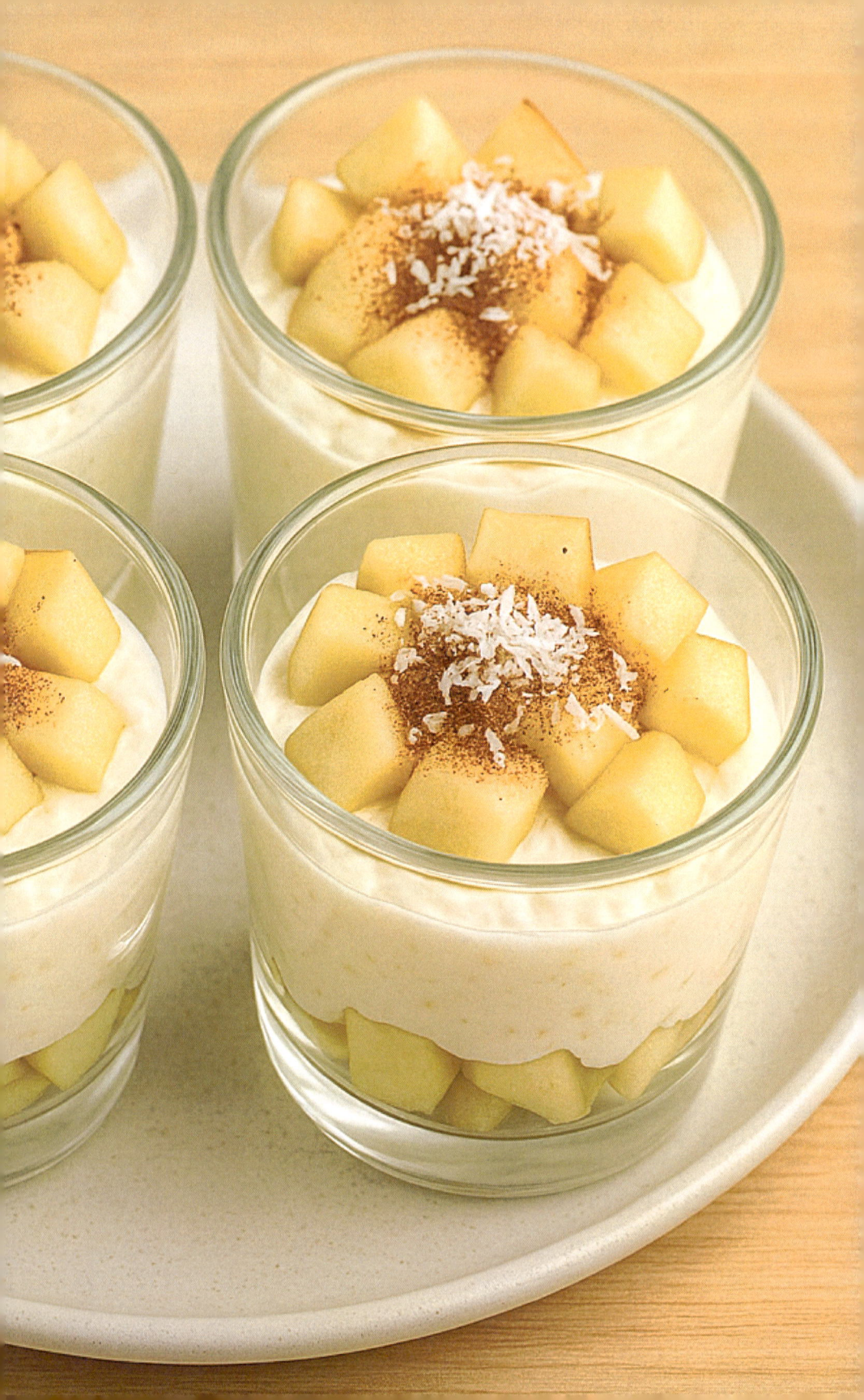

Apfel Quark Cups (German)

Quark is a very soft, slightly tart cheese popular in Germany and other parts of Europe. You can find it in specialty stores, but Greek yogurt will work as well. If you want to top your cups with something other than graham crackers, try chocolate chips or coconut.

Ingredients:
2 medium apples (peeled and chopped small)
1 tablespoon butter or margarine
1 tablespoon sugar (white or brown)
½ teaspoon cinnamon
250g (about 1 cup) quark (or use Greek yogurt if quark isn't available)
2 tablespoons honey or maple syrup
1 teaspoon vanilla extract (optional)
4 crushed shortbread cookies or graham crackers (for topping)

Tools You'll Need:
A frying pan
A mixing bowl
A spoon
Measuring spoons
4 small cups or bowls

Step-by-Step Instructions:

1 Cook the apples.
Put the butter in a frying pan on medium heat. Add the chopped apples, sugar, and cinnamon. Stir often for 5–7 minutes, until apples are soft. Turn off the heat. Let the apples cool a little.

2 Mix the quark filling.
In a bowl, add the quark, honey, and vanilla. Stir until it's smooth.

3 Make the dessert cups.
In each small cup or bowl, put a spoonful of quark mix. Add a spoonful of the cooked apples. Repeat until the cup is full (about 2 layers of each). Sprinkle crushed cookies on top.

4 Serve or chill.
Eat right away, or put in the fridge for later. It tastes even better cold!

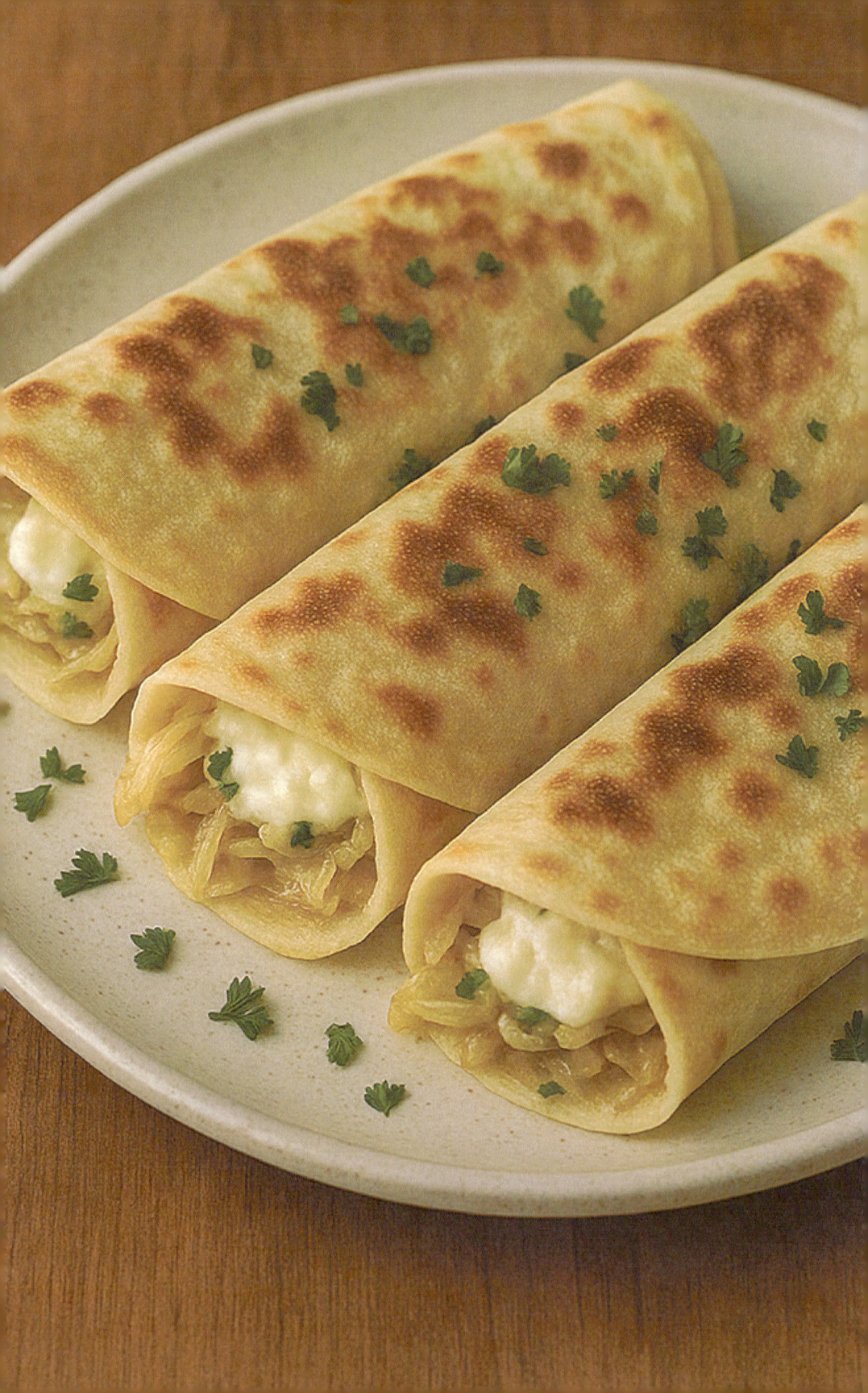

Azerbaijani Cheese Qutab Wraps

Azerbaijan is a small country in the Caucasus region bordering Russia, Georgia, Armenia, and Iran. "Qutab" wraps are similar to crepes and are usually served either for breakfast or as a snack.

Ingredients:
(Makes 2 wraps)
2 soft flour tortillas (8-inch)
½ cup grated mozzarella or feta cheese (or mix!)
1 tablespoon chopped fresh herbs (parsley, mint, or dill) – or 1 tsp dried herbs
1 tablespoon plain yogurt (for dipping, optional)
1 teaspoon oil or butter (for cooking)

Tools You'll Need:
Frying pan
Spatula
Butter knife or spoon
Plate
Measuring spoon

Step-by-Step Instructions:

1 Make the Filling
In a small bowl, mix the cheese and herbs together with a spoon.

2 Fill the Tortillas
Lay each tortilla flat on a plate. Put half the cheese mix on one side of each tortilla. Fold the other half over to make a half-moon shape. Press gently.

3 Cook the Qutab Wraps
Heat a little oil or butter in the frying pan on medium. Place one folded tortilla in the pan. Cook for 2–3 minutes on each side until golden and the cheese melts. Repeat with the second one.

4 Serve and Dip
Place on a plate. Let cool slightly, then cut in half (if you like). Serve with a little plain yogurt for dipping.

Tips for Accessibility:
Use pre-shredded cheese and pre-cut herbs.

Dried herbs work just as well for ease.

If stovetop use is tricky, you can microwave the folded tortilla for 45–60 seconds instead.

Let the person press and fold the wrap—it's a satisfying, hands-on step!

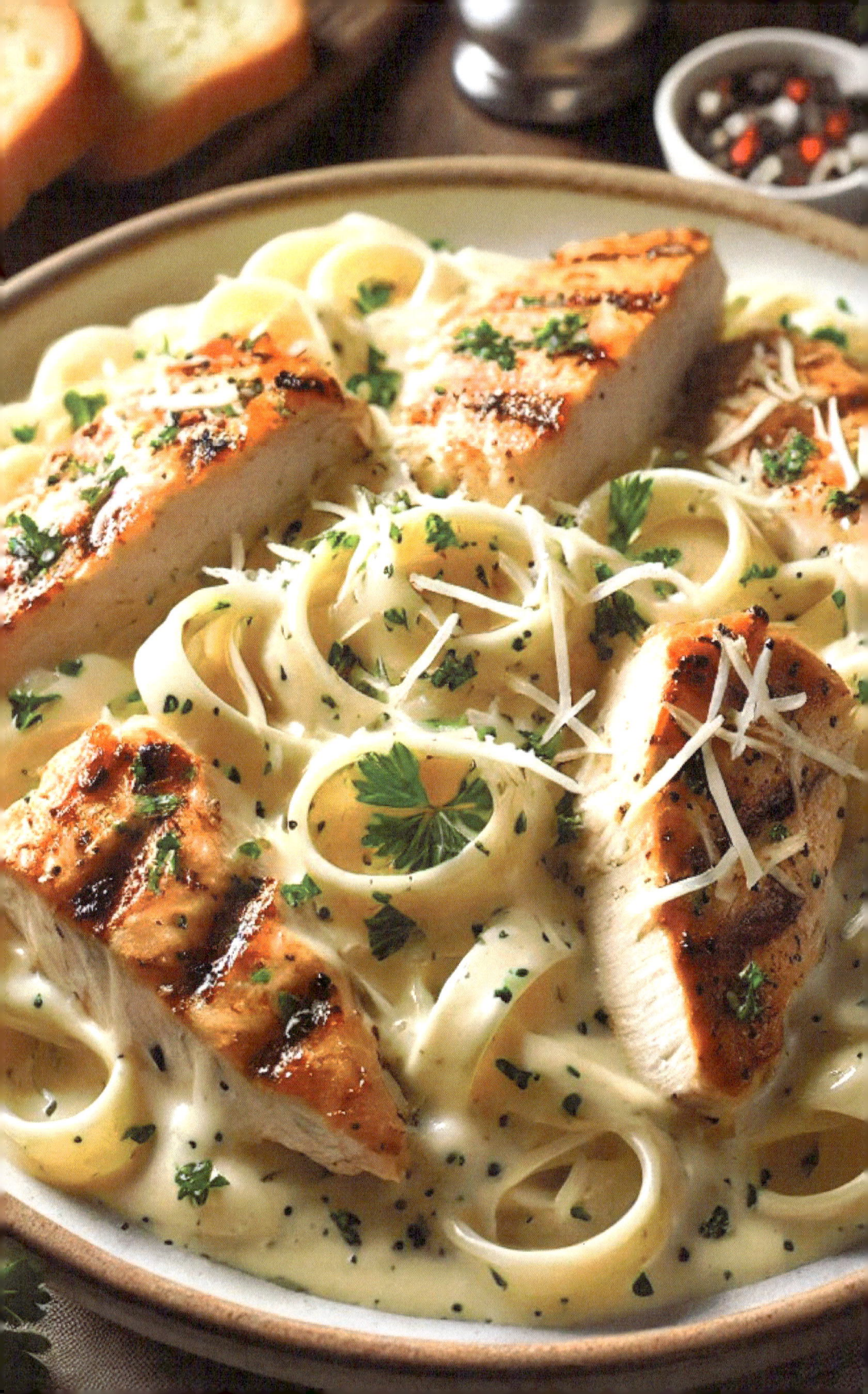

Easy Chicken Pasta Alfredo

Pasta Alfredo is creamy and indulgent, and this recipe is an easy way to get the ultimate comfort meal on the table in no time. I recommend topping with shredded Parmesan cheese and serving with some garlic bread.

Ingredients:
1 pound of boneless, skinless chicken breasts
1 jar of Alfredo sauce
1 box of linguini noodles
1 small onion (chopped)
2 garlic cloves (chopped)
1 Tablespoon olive oil
Salt to taste
Optional: ¼ cup shredded Parmesan cheese

Tools You'll Need:
Medium pot
Large skillet
Measuring cups and spoons
Colander

Step-by-Step Instructions:

1 Make your Linguini.
   Add water to a medium pot and bring to a boil. Add a pinch of salt and a teaspoon of oil, and then add the linguini noodles and cook according to package instructions. Drain in a colander and set aside.

2 Cook your chicken.
   In a large skillet, heat a tablespoon of olive oil over medium heat. Add the garlic and cook, stirring frequently, until fragrant. Add onion and cook for an additional minute. Add your chicken and cook, flipping it occasionally, until it is browned.

3 Finish your Alfredo sauce.
   Add your Alfredo sauce to the skillet with your chicken. Add salt and pepper to taste, then bring to a boil. Once it comes to a boil, add your linguini noodles and simmer on low for 10 minutes.

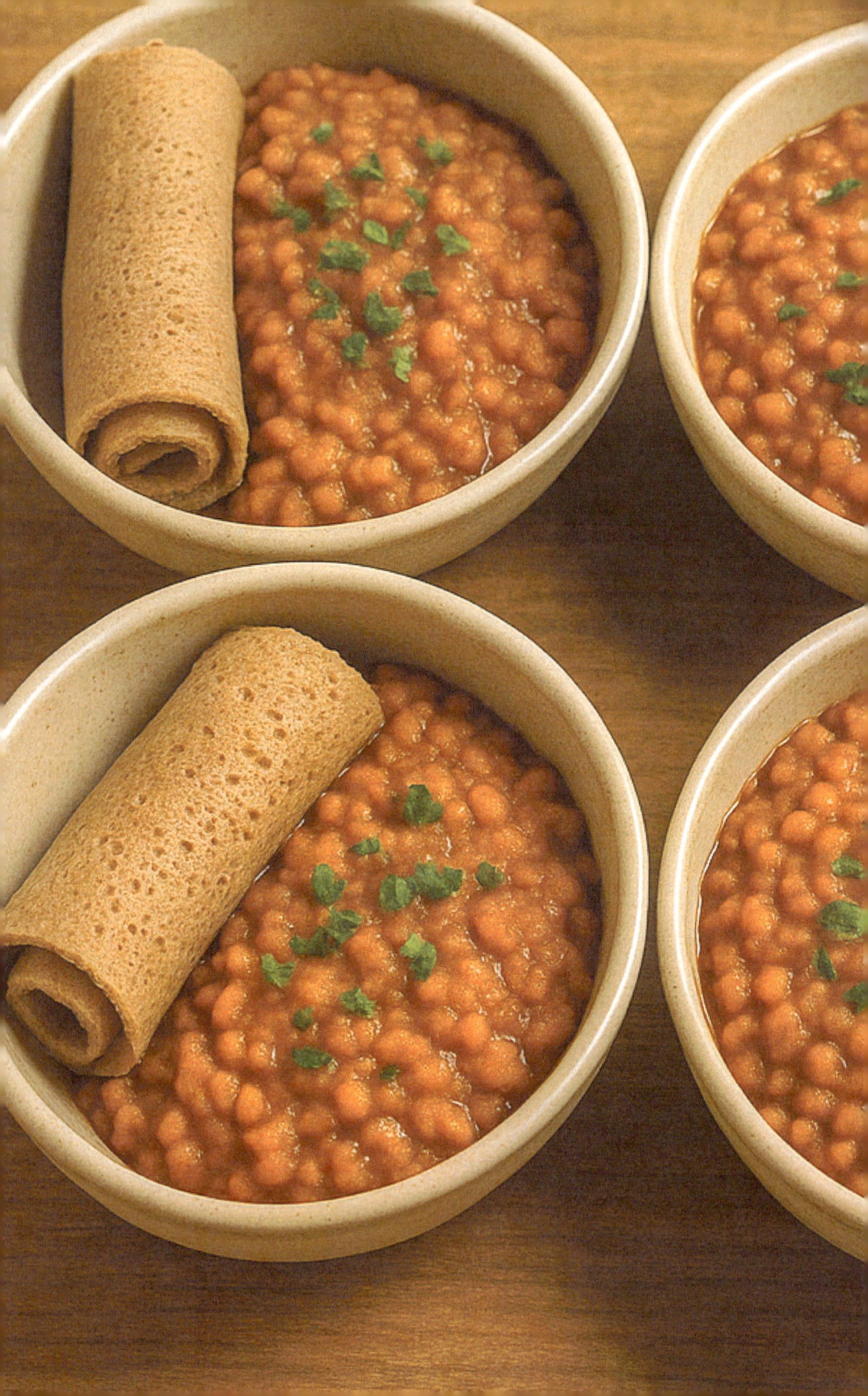

Ethiopian Lentil Bowls with Injera Scoops

A warm, flavorful lentil stew served with torn pieces of soft injera (similar to pita bread) for scooping instead of a fork or spoon. Lentils are a staple of the Ethiopian diet. It's easier just to use canned lentils, but if you have dried red lentils, just make sure you soak them overnight before cooking them for optimal digestion.

Ingredients:
(Makes 2 servings)
1 cup cooked lentils (canned or pre-cooked)
½ cup canned diced tomatoes
½ teaspoon berbere spice blend (or use a mix of paprika and a pinch of chili powder)
1 tablespoon oil or butter
¼ teaspoon garlic powder
Salt to taste
2 small injera (store-bought or pre-made) – or use soft tortillas if unavailable
Optional: a spoonful of plain yogurt on top

Tools You'll Need:
Pan or saucepan
Spoon for stirring
Bowl and spoon for eating

Tips for Accessibility:
Use canned lentils to skip boiling.

No knives or cutting needed.

Injera is soft, stretchy, and easy to tear—great for sensory-friendly eating.

Simple stirring steps and warm colors/smells create an enjoyable experience.

Everything is soft and scoopable—no chewing challenges.

Step-by-Step Instructions:

1 **Warm the oil and spices.**
In a saucepan, add oil. Sprinkle in berbere spice and garlic powder. Stir gently on low heat for 1 minute to release the aroma.

2 **Add lentils and tomatoes.**
Add lentils and canned tomatoes (with a little of the juice). Stir everything together.

3 **Simmer and soften.**
Cook on medium heat for 5–10 minutes, stirring occasionally, until it thickens. Add a pinch of salt to taste.

4 **Serve with Injera.**
Spoon the warm lentil stew into a bowl. Tear soft injera into pieces and place on the side or directly on top.

5 **Scoop and enjoy.**
Use pieces of injera to scoop the lentils. Top with yogurt if you like it creamy!

Israeli Egg Pita Pockets

A warm pita stuffed with eggs, veggies, and a creamy tahini-yogurt drizzle. This is a traditional Israeli breakfast, usually served with Israeli coffee. Think of it as a Middle Eastern twist on the breakfast burrito!

Ingredients:
(Makes 2 pita pockets)
2 pita breads (store-bought is perfect)
2 eggs
½ cucumber (chopped small)
1 small tomato (chopped small)
2 tablespoons plain yogurt
1 tablespoon tahini (sesame paste – optional)
1 teaspoon lemon juice or a splash of water
A pinch of salt

Optional Add-ins:
A sprinkle of za'atar or chopped parsley
A spoonful of hummus inside the pita
A few olives on the side

Tools You'll Need:
Frying pan
Spatula
Small bowl and spoon
Knife (or pre-chopped veggies)
Plate

Step-by-Step Instructions:

1 **Scramble the eggs.**
Heat the pan on medium. Crack the eggs into a bowl, mix with a fork, then pour into the pan. Stir gently until cooked. Turn off the heat.

2 **Chop the veggies.**
Cut the cucumber and tomato into small pieces. If that's tricky, you can ask someone to help or use pre-chopped veggies.

3 **Make the sauce.**
In a small bowl, mix yogurt, tahini, lemon juice (or water), and a pinch of salt. Stir until smooth and creamy.

4 **Warm the pitas.**
You can warm the pitas in the pan for 30 seconds on each side or microwave them for 10–15 seconds to make them soft.

5 **Fill the pockets.**
Cut each pita in half to make a pocket. Carefully open and fill each half with scrambled eggs, chopped veggies, and a spoonful of yogurt sauce.

6 Eat and enjoy.

Serve on a plate with extra sauce or hummus on the side. Pick it up with your hands—no fork needed!

Tips for Accessibility:

You can prepare the sauce ahead of time—it lasts a few days in the fridge.

If pita is hard to open, wrap it in a damp paper towel and microwave for 15 seconds to soften.

Great for visual learners: use photos or color-coded ingredient bowls!

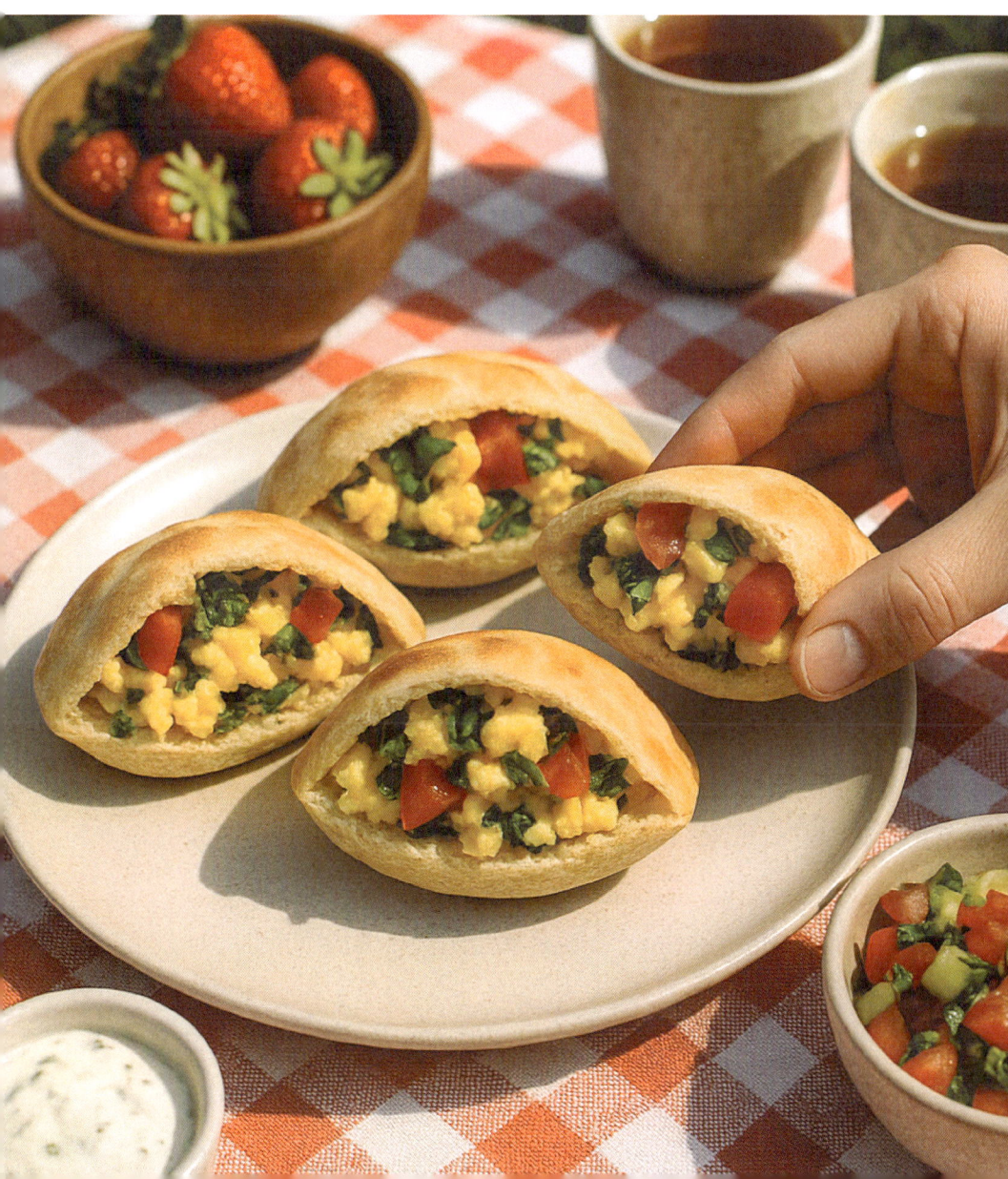

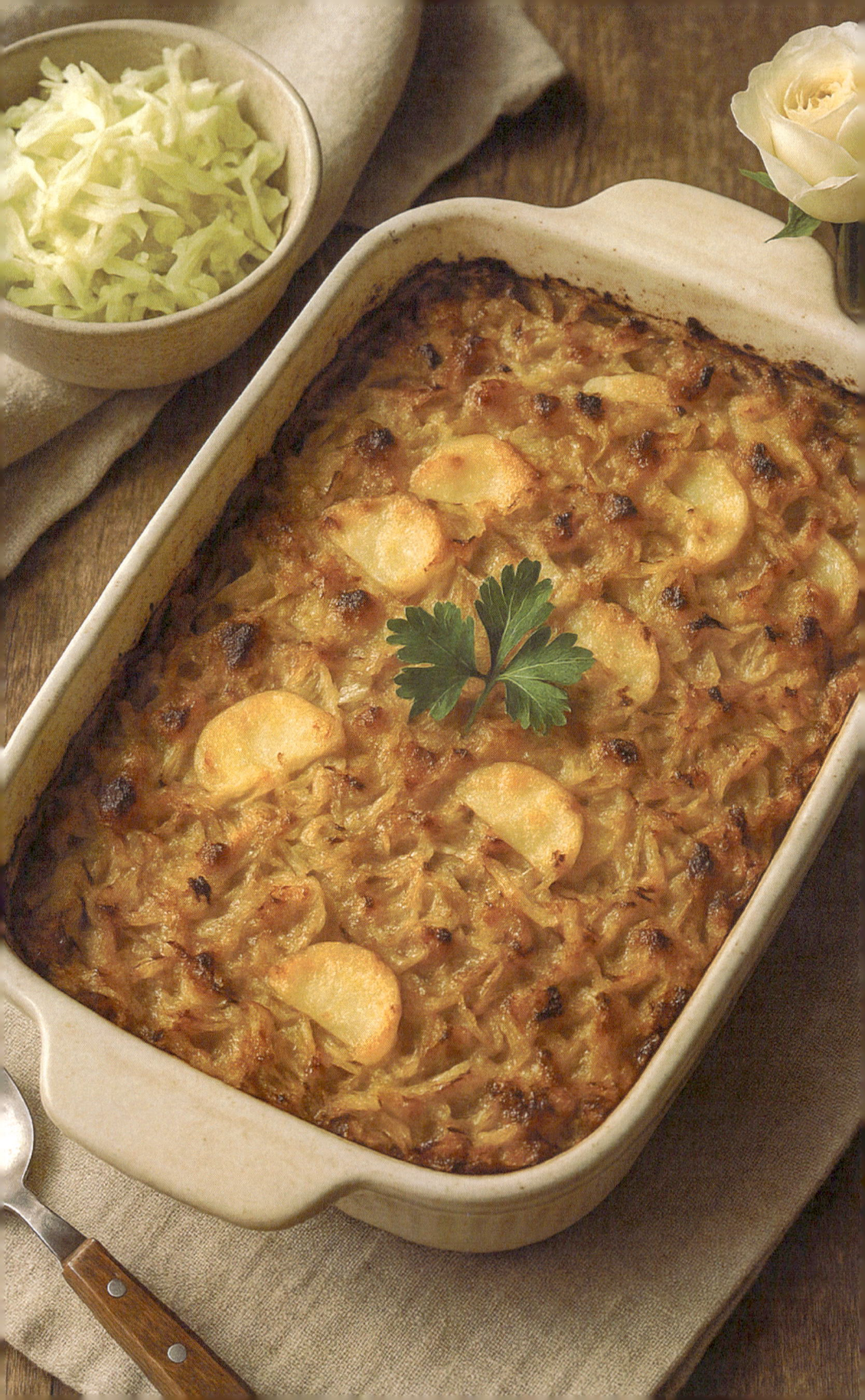

Ukrainian Cabbage & Potato Bake

A soft, cozy casserole with mashed potatoes, sautéed cabbage, and a hint of dill—just stir, layer, and bake! Cabbage is used often in Eastern European cuisine, and you'll find it has a great flavor when baked, which is complemented by the buttery mashed potatoes.

Ingredients:

2 cups mashed potatoes (use instant, leftover, or store-bought)
1½ cups shredded cabbage (fresh or packaged coleslaw mix)
1 tablespoon butter or oil
½ teaspoon dried dill (or parsley)
½ teaspoon onion powder
Salt and pepper to taste
Optional: ½ cup shredded cheese for the top
Optional: 2 tablespoons sour cream for serving

Tools You'll Need:

Frying pan or saucepan
Mixing bowl
Spoon
Baking dish (small casserole or 8x8 pan)
Oven or toaster oven

Step-by-Step Instructions:

1 **Cook the cabbage.**
In a pan, heat butter or oil over medium heat. Add the cabbage, onion powder, dill, and a pinch of salt. Stir and cook for 5–7 minutes until soft. Turn off the heat and let it cool for a few minutes.

2 Preheat oven.
Set your oven or toaster oven to 180°C (350°F).

3 Layer the casserole.
In a greased baking dish, spread half the mashed potatoes.
Spoon all the cooked cabbage over the potatoes.
Add the rest of the mashed potatoes on top and smooth them out.
Sprinkle cheese on top (if using).

4 Bake.
Bake for 20–25 minutes until warm and slightly golden on top. Let cool for 5 minutes.

5 Serve.
Scoop into bowls and top with a dollop of sour cream if you like. Eat warm with a spoon or fork.

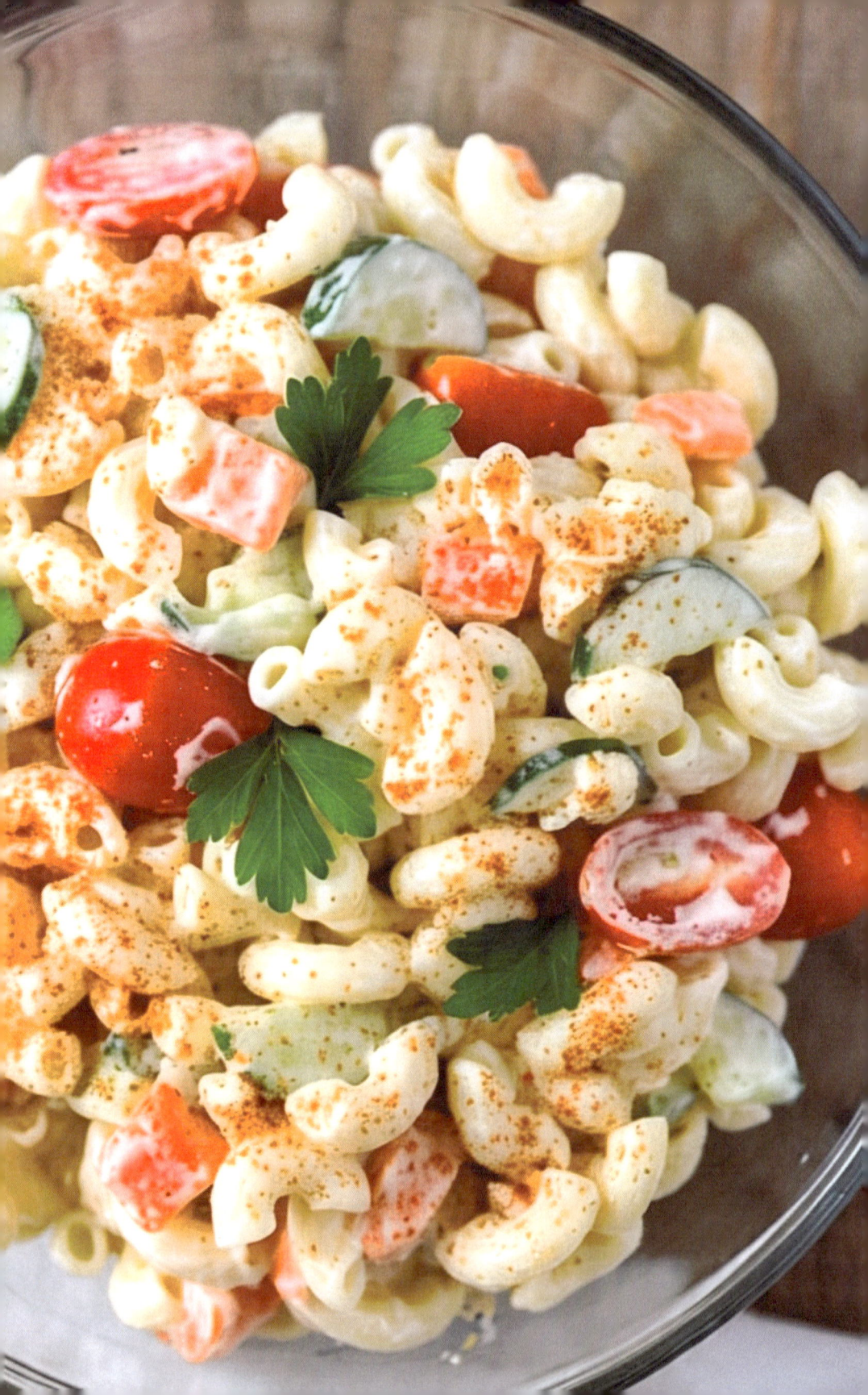

Elbow Pasta Salad

Pasta salad is a great make-ahead option for busy weeks or for a surprise dinner party. This one is vegetarian, with some beans for protein. I use garbanzo beans, but any type of bean you have on hand will work.

Ingredients:
3 cups of elbow pasta
1 can of mixed vegetables
1 can of garbanzo beans
3 tablespoons light mayonnaise
1 teaspoon garlic powder
Salt and pepper to taste

Tools You'll Need:
Medium pot
Measuring cups and spoons
Spatula or wooden spoon
Large bowl
Colander

Step-by-Step Instructions:

1 Boil your pasta.
   In a medium pot filled with water, bring to a boil over medium-high heat, then add pasta and cook according to package directions. Drain in a colander and set aside to cool.

2 Assemble your pasta salad.
   In a large bowl, add your can of mixed vegetables, garbanzo beans, garlic powder, and pasta. Add in the mayonnaise and mix everything together. Season to taste with salt and pepper.

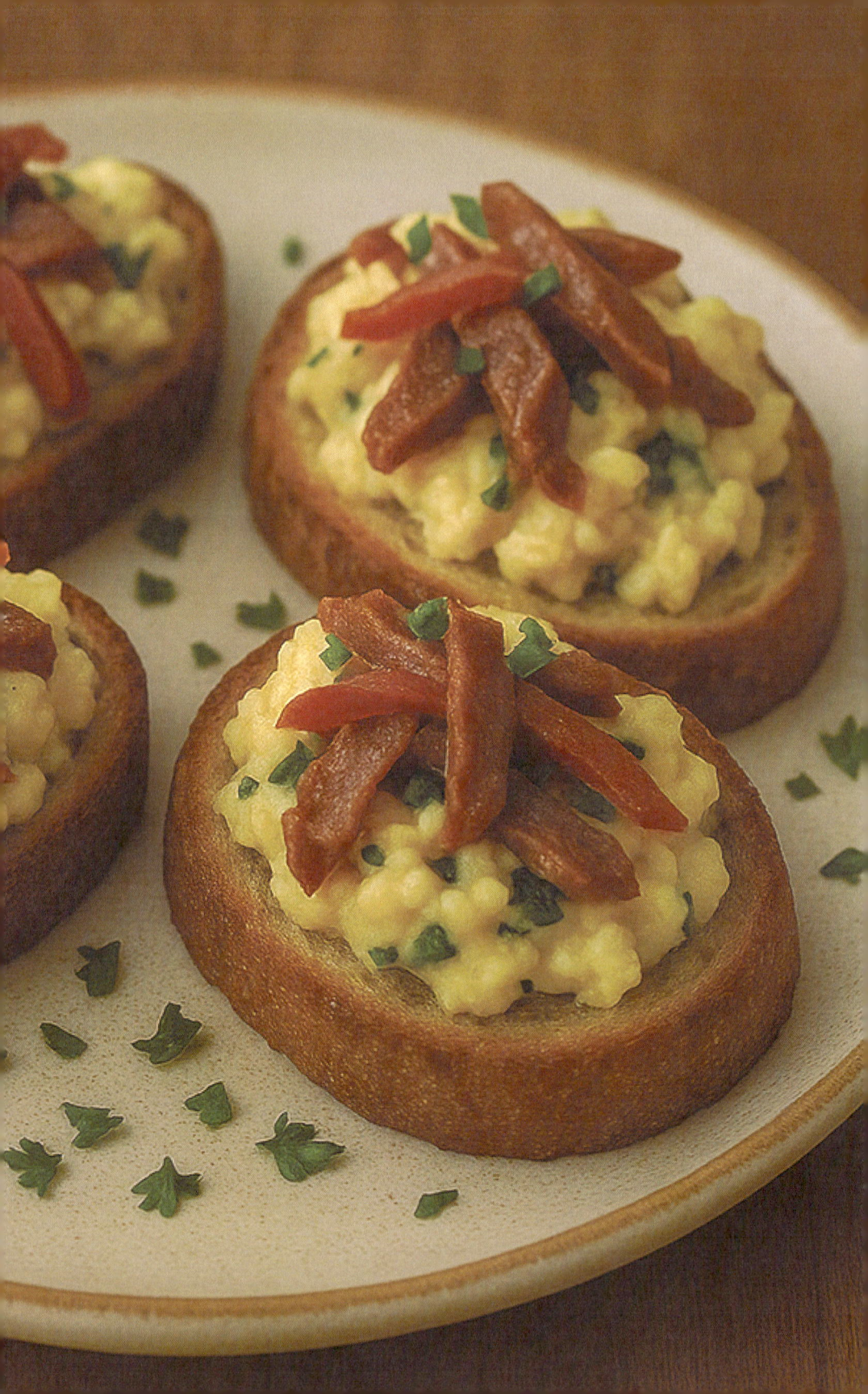

Hungarian Breakfast Toasties

A warm open-faced sandwich with eggs, paprika, and melted cheese—and particularly tasty using Hungarian paprika, although smoked paprika will work as well. I like to add leftover sausage or bacon to mine, but leftover veggies or even avocado work too.

Ingredients:
Makes 4 toasties
4 slices of bread (any kind you like)
2 eggs
½ cup shredded cheese (like mozzarella or cheddar)
2 tablespoons sour cream
½ teaspoon sweet Hungarian paprika
A pinch of salt
Optional: chopped green pepper or cooked sausage pieces

Tools You'll Need:
Bowl
Spoon or fork
Toaster oven or oven
Baking tray (with foil or baking paper)

Step-by-Step Instructions:

1 **Make the egg spread.**
In a bowl, crack the eggs. Add sour cream, paprika, and a pinch of salt. Mix it all together with a fork until smooth.

2 **Add cheese.**
Stir the shredded cheese into the egg mixture. If using sausage or green pepper, add a little now, too.

3 **Prepare the bread.**
Put the slices of bread on a baking tray. Spoon the egg mixture evenly on top of each slice.

4 **Bake the toasties.**
Put the tray in the oven or toaster oven. Bake at 180°C (350°F) for 10–12 minutes, or until the egg is cooked and the cheese is melted.

5 **Cool and serve.**
Let cool for 2 minutes, then serve warm. It can be eaten with fingers or a fork and knife.

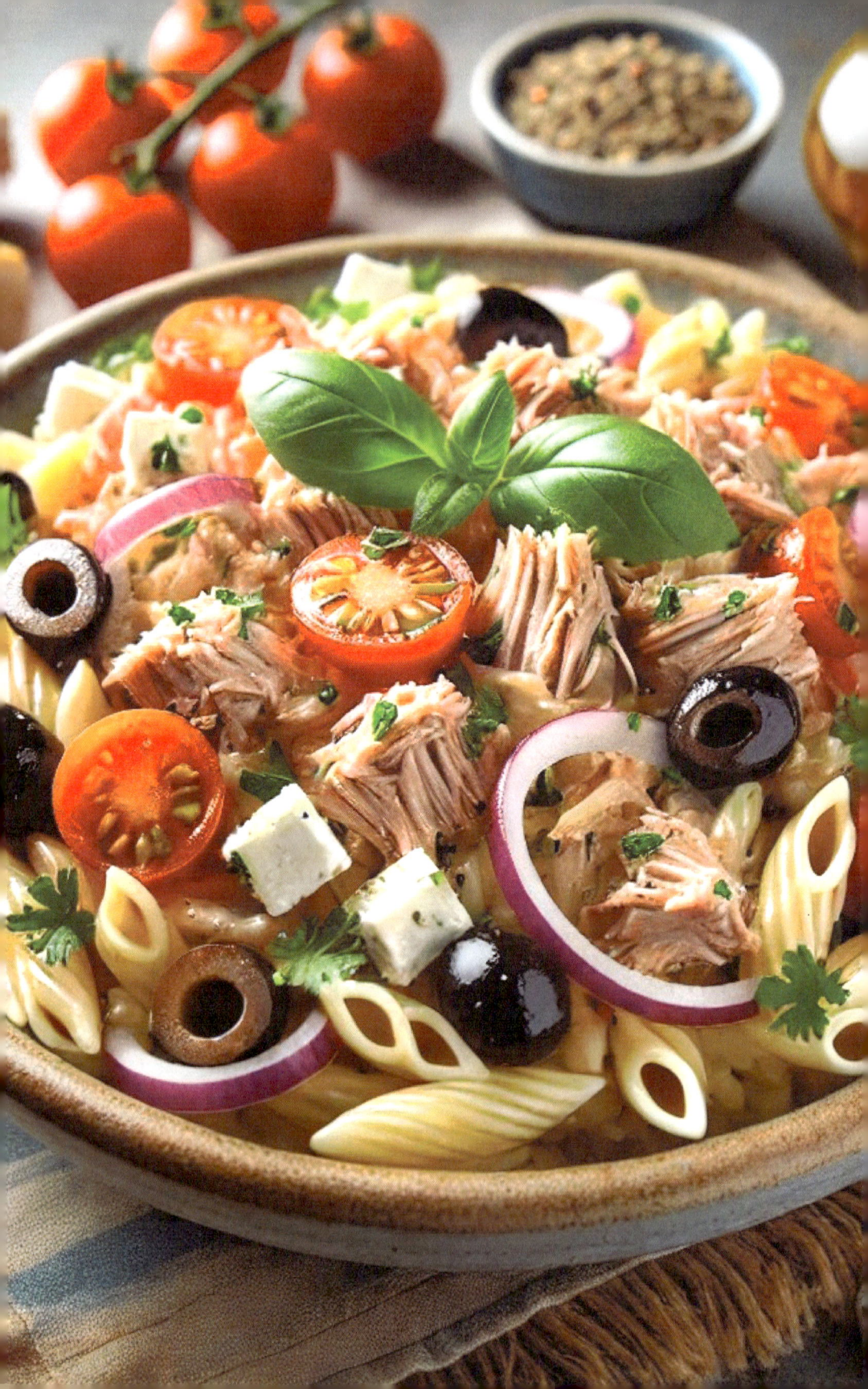

Italian Orzo Tuna Salad

An Italian twist on a staple lunch offering. Orzo handles the dressing well, but if you need to use another pasta that you have on hand, it should work fine. Try to stick to shaped pasta like spirals or bow-tie so it doesn't get too soggy.

Ingredients:
1 package of orzo (or your preferred pasta)
1 10-ounce can of tuna, drained
1 small jar of sun dried tomatoes, chopped (or use fresh tomatoes, but cut out the seeds)
½ red onion (coarsely chopped)
A handful of fresh spinach or other leafy greens
⅓ cup toasted pine nuts
1 handful fresh basil (chopped)
½ cup Italian vinaigrette salad dressing
⅓ cup grated Parmesan
Salt and pepper to taste

Tools You'll Need:
Medium pot
Spoon
Measuring cups and spoons
Large bowl
Colander

Step-by-Step Instructions:

1 Cook your pasta.
  Using a medium pot and lightly salted water, cook your pasta according to package directions. Drain and then toss with tuna in a large bowl.

2 Mix the remaining ingredients.
  Mix in the sun dried tomatoes, basil, onion, and spinach with the tuna and pasta. Season to taste with salt and pepper and sprinkle on Parmesan before serving.

Italian Meatballs and Fettuccine

Homemade meatballs just taste better than frozen ones, but if you want to save some time, just use frozen, and once cooked, simply mix them in with the cooked noodles and marinara sauce. You can also use whichever type of noodles you have on hand.

Ingredients:

1 pound ground turkey or beef
1 bag of fettuccine noodles (or whichever pasta you prefer)
½ cup breadcrumbs
2 eggs
1 tablespoon Italian seasoning
1 tablespoon parsley (fresh or dried)
1 tsp dried oregano
1 tsp dried basil
½ cup parmesan cheese (grated)
1 clove chopped garlic
1 tsp salt
1 tsp red pepper flakes
1 jar of marinara sauce
1 zucchini (diced)
½ cup onion (diced)

Tools You'll Need:

Medium baking dish
Spoon
Measuring cups and spoons
Knife
1 large sauce pot
1 large bowl
Colander

Tips for Accessibility:

Use frozen meatballs instead of making them.

Instead of making sauce, find one in a flavor you like and heat it on the stovetop before adding it to pasta and meatballs.

Step-by-Step Instructions:

1 Heat oven to 350 degrees.
   While the oven heats, use a large pot of boiling salted water to cook your fettuccine (or other noodles) according to package instructions. Drain pasta in colander and set aside.

2 Prepare meatballs.
   In a large bowl, combine the meat with breadcrumbs, Italian seasoning, parsley, parmesan, eggs, garlic, salt, and red pepper flakes. Mix with your hands until just combined (don't over mix!) and then use wet hands to form into 16 1-inch-sized meatballs.

3 Bake meatballs.
   Spray a large baking dish with Pam (or lightly coat with oil) and place the meatballs inside, spaced slightly apart. Place in the oven and cook, turning once or twice, until brown on all sides, about 10-12 minutes. Transfer meatballs to a plate.

4 Make your sauce.

In a medium-sized saucepan on medium heat, add olive oil and cook onions and zucchini until soft, about five minutes. Add marinara sauce, basil, and oregano and stir. Pour meatballs into the saucepan, lower the heat, and simmer covered for five minutes.

5 Plate your pasta.

Place pasta in individual bowls and top with meatballs and sauce. Top with parmesan before serving.

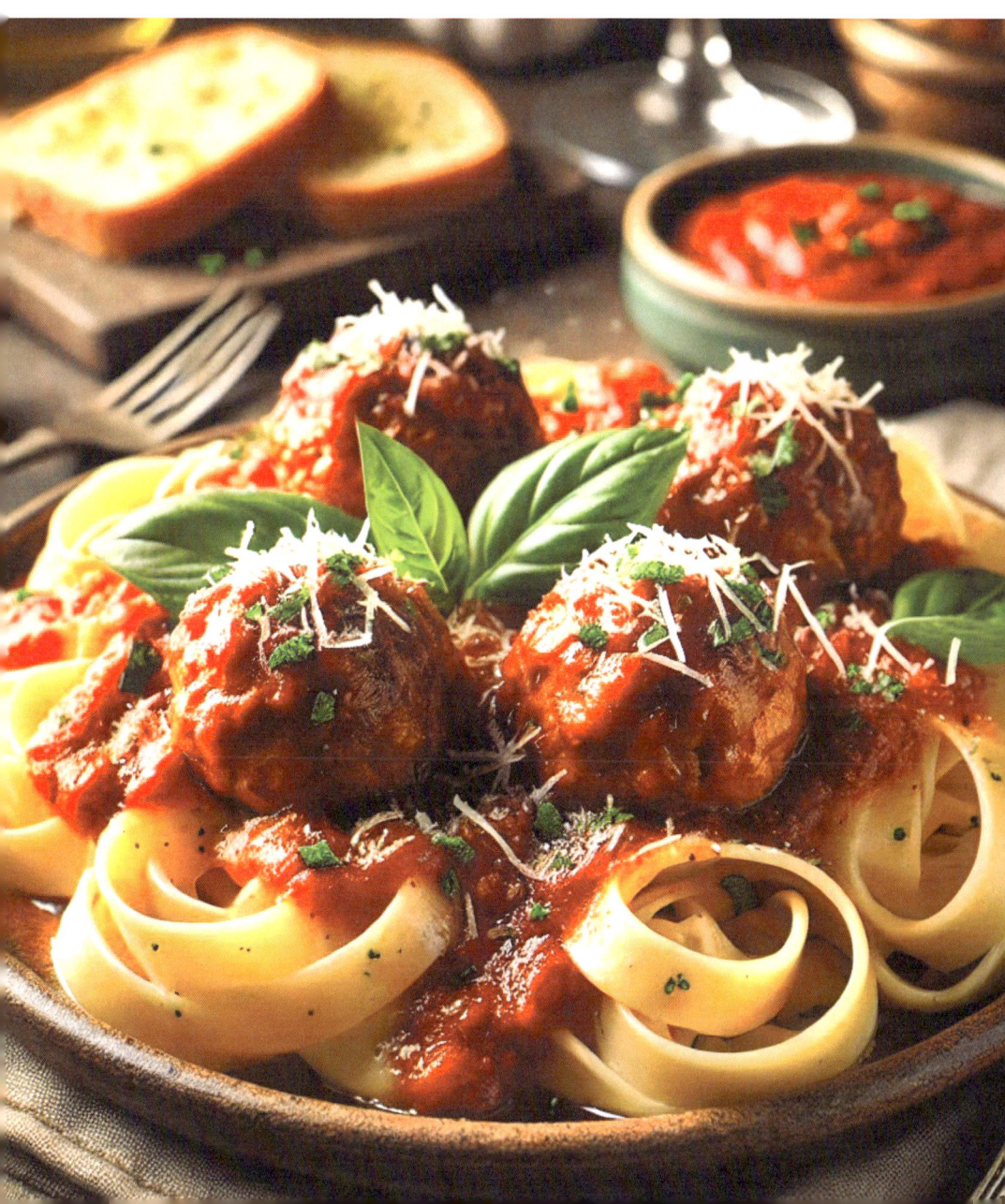

Italian Red Rose Pasta from San Marino

My great-grandfather lived in San Marino, Italy. I love making this traditional Italian dish and thinking about my Italian ancestors making it all those years ago. It tastes best when you use Prosciutto, but any thinly sliced meat will work in a pinch. The rich Béchamel sauce is one you'll never forget.

Ingredients:

8 pieces of lasagna pasta noodles
¾ pound of Prosciutto sliced thin (you can also use sliced ham, bacon, turkey or chicken)
1 ⅓ cup Fontina cheese (thinly sliced)
12 fresh basil leaves
1 ½ cups marinara sauce
Optional: Grated Parmesan cheese for topping

For the Béchamel Sauce:

3 tablespoons all-purpose flour
2 tablespoons butter
1 ½ cups whole milk
⅛ teaspoon grated nutmeg
2 tablespoons Parmesan cheese (grated)
Salt to taste

Tools You'll Need:

Small saucepan
Spoon
Whisk
Measuring cups and spoons
Medium pot
Slotted spoon
Large baking dish

Step-by-Step Instructions:

1 Make the béchamel sauce.
Whisk the milk and flour together in a small saucepan. Add the butter and heat the pan over moderate to high heat. Keep whisking until the sauce thickens. Season with salt, nutmeg, and the two tablespoons of Parmesan cheese, then turn off the heat and let sit.

2 Prepare your lasagna noodles.
Cook lasagna pieces in a large pot of boiling, salted water for 10 minutes. Remove noodles carefully with a slotted spoon and place on kitchen towels. Turn them over to dry on both sides, then arrange them on a plate or cutting board.

3 Preheat the oven to 325 degrees.
Coat the bottom of a large baking dish with marinara sauce.

4 Prepare lasagna noodles.

On each lasagna piece, spread a layer of béchamel sauce, then sprinkle with Parmesan cheese and place slices of prosciutto, basil, and Fontina cheese on top. Roll each lasagna piece into a tight cylinder. Place them close together, cut side up, in the baking dish.

5 Cook for 10 minutes, until the cheese melts and the cylinder is lightly browned. Sprinkle with additional Parmesan if desired and serve.

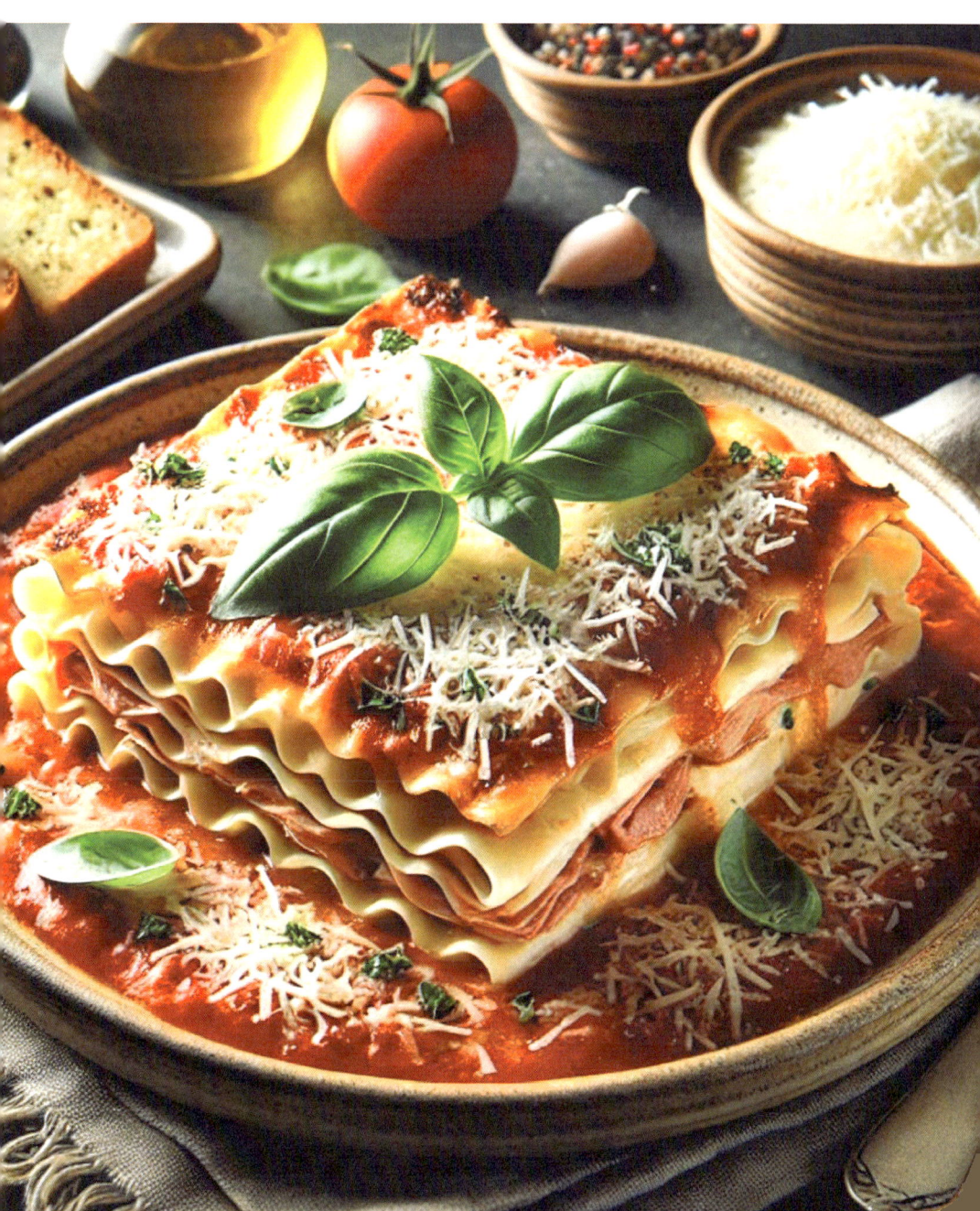

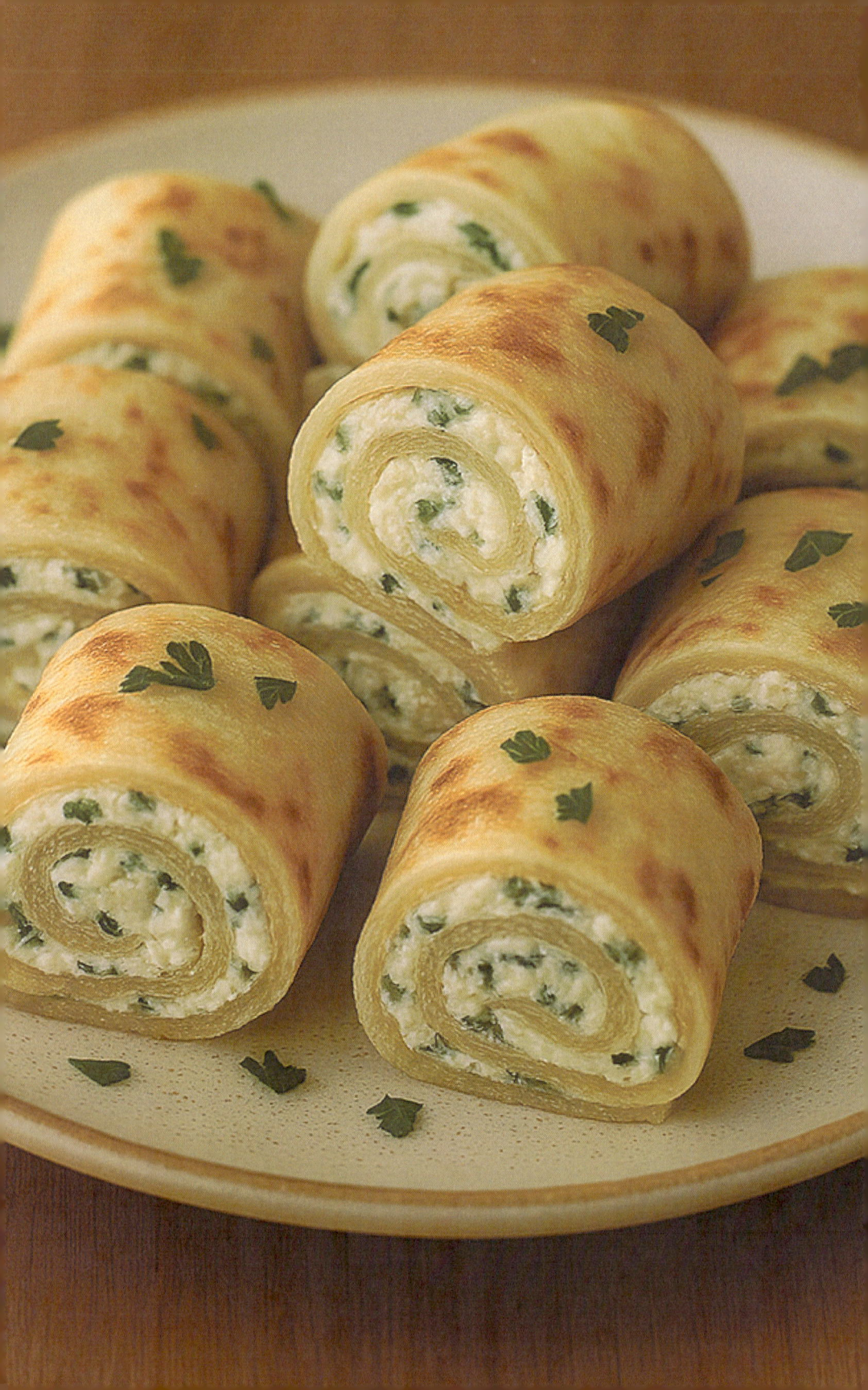

Lazy Blini Roll-Ups

A sweet twist on Russian blini (thin pancakes), turned into soft dessert rolls with jam and creamy filling. "Lazy" because it's super easy!

Ingredients:
Makes 4 roll-ups
4 store-bought crepes or thin pancakes (or use ready-made blini if available)
½ cup plain cream cheese or ricotta (for soft texture)
2 tablespoons sugar or honey
½ teaspoon vanilla (optional)
¼ cup fruit jam (strawberry, raspberry, or apricot – Russian favorites!)
A dusting of powdered sugar (optional, for topping)

Tools You'll Need:
Butter knife or spoon
Small bowl
Plate
Fork (optional)

Tips for Accessibility:
Use plastic knives or spoons for safe spreading.

Let the person choose their favorite jam for a fun decision-making step.

Each roll can be made one at a time to avoid overwhelm.

No cooking involved—just assembling!

Step-by-Step Instructions:

1 **Make the creamy filling.**
In a small bowl, mix the cream cheese (or ricotta) with sugar or honey. Add vanilla if using. Stir until smooth.

2 **Lay out the pancakes.**
Place one pancake flat on a plate or clean surface.

3 **Spread and roll.**
Spread a thin layer of jam on the pancake, then add a spoonful of the cream mixture on top. Gently spread it too. Roll up the pancake like a soft burrito or jelly roll.

4 **Repeat and slice.**
Do the same for all four pancakes. You can leave them whole or slice each into 2–3 smaller pieces to make cute dessert rolls.

5 **Dust and serve.**
Sprinkle a little powdered sugar on top if you like. Eat with fingers or a fork. Tastes great warm or cold!

Meat Lasagna

One of my favorite things about cooking is that it can transport you to places you might not be able to afford to travel to. This is why I love making Italian recipes, so I can pretend I am traveling there myself. This meat lasagna is one of those great traditional Italian dishes that are worth the effort. You can make this with lean turkey and ground beef if that's what you have on hand, but when you use ground Italian sausage in place of the turkey, the flavors really pop!

Ingredients:

1 package lasagna noodles, uncooked
1 pound ground beef
1 pound ground Italian sausage
4 cups ricotta cheese
1 cup grated Parmesan cheese
2 cups mozzarella cheese (shredded)
2 cups fresh spinach, lightly packed and roughly chopped
1 medium onion, finely chopped
2 cloves garlic, finely chopped
2 tablespoons olive oil
1 teaspoon dried oregano
1 teaspoon dried basil
Optional: pinch of red pepper flakes

Tools You'll Need:

Large pot
Dish towel
Medium saucepan
Medium bowl
Measuring cups and spoons
Wooden spoon
Large baking dish
Colander

Step-by-Step Instructions:

1 **Preheat oven to 350 degrees F and cook your lasagna noodles.**
Fill a large pot with water and add 1 tablespoon salt and 2 tablespoons olive oil. Bring to a boil and add your pasta. Cook for 10 minutes, then drain. Spread lasagna noodles on a clean dish towel to dry.

2 **Cook your meat mixture.**
In a medium saucepan, sauté the beef and sausage together, crumbling with a wooden spoon, until the beef is no longer pink and cooked through. Add chopped onion, garlic, and oregano. Continue sautéing for another four minutes until the sausage is cooked through. Add your marinara sauce to the meat mixture, turn off the heat, and set aside.

3 **Make your ricotta filling.**
In a medium bowl, blend ricotta cheese, ½ cup of the grated Parmesan cheese, and the spinach. Set aside.

4 Assemble your lasagna in an oven-safe baking dish.

Coat the baking dish with 1 cup of the meat mixture. Line a pan with lasagna noodles to form one layer. Spread ½ of the ricotta cheese mixture on top of the noodles. Spread ½ of the meat sauce, 1 cup of mozzarella, and ¼ cup Parmesan cheese over the meat. That is one layer. Repeat this process, starting with the noodle layer, until you're out of noodles, then sprinkle red pepper flakes and any remaining cheese on top.

5 Bake in the oven for 45 minutes until hot and bubbly.

Remove carefully and let stand 10 minutes before slicing and serving.

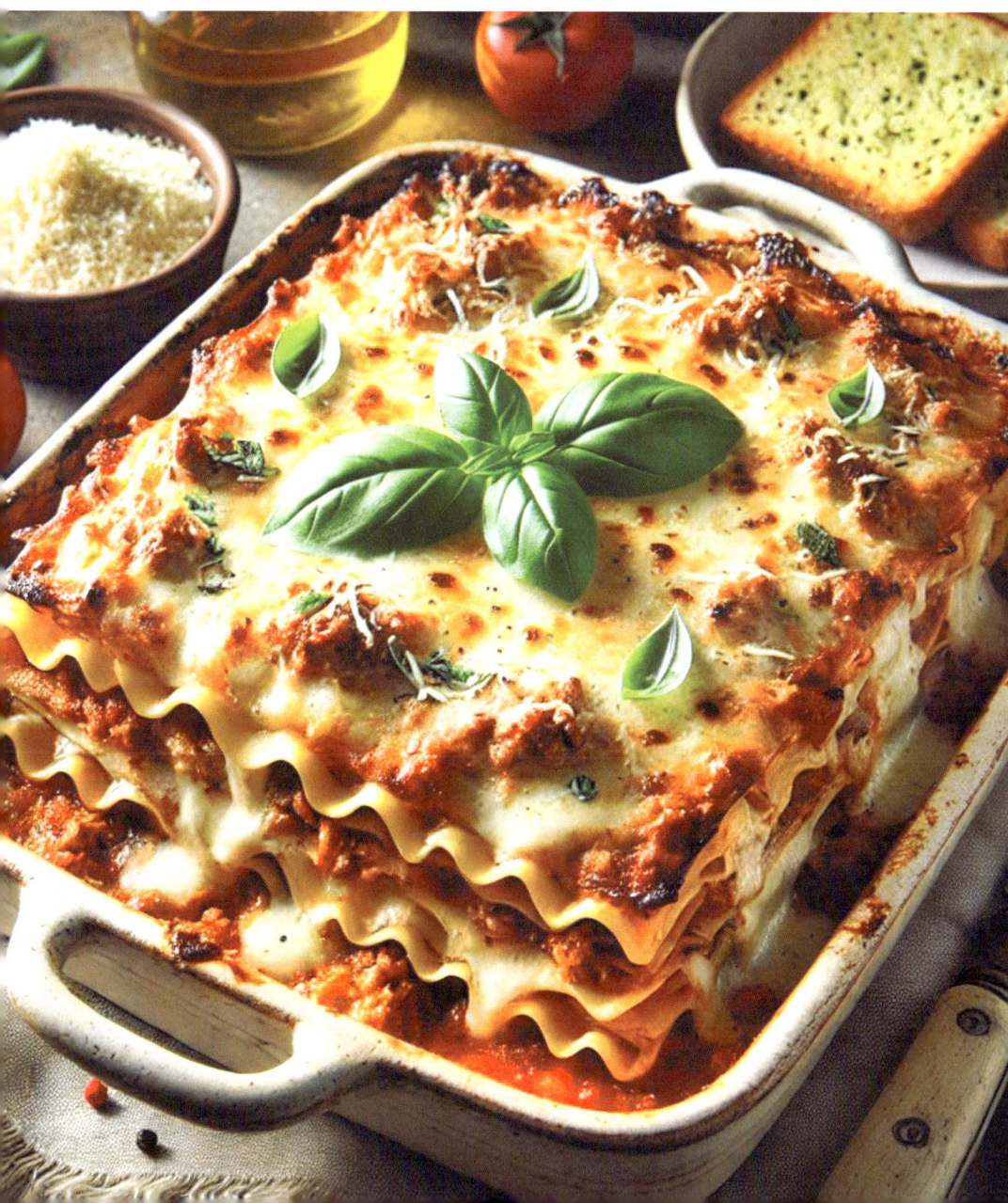

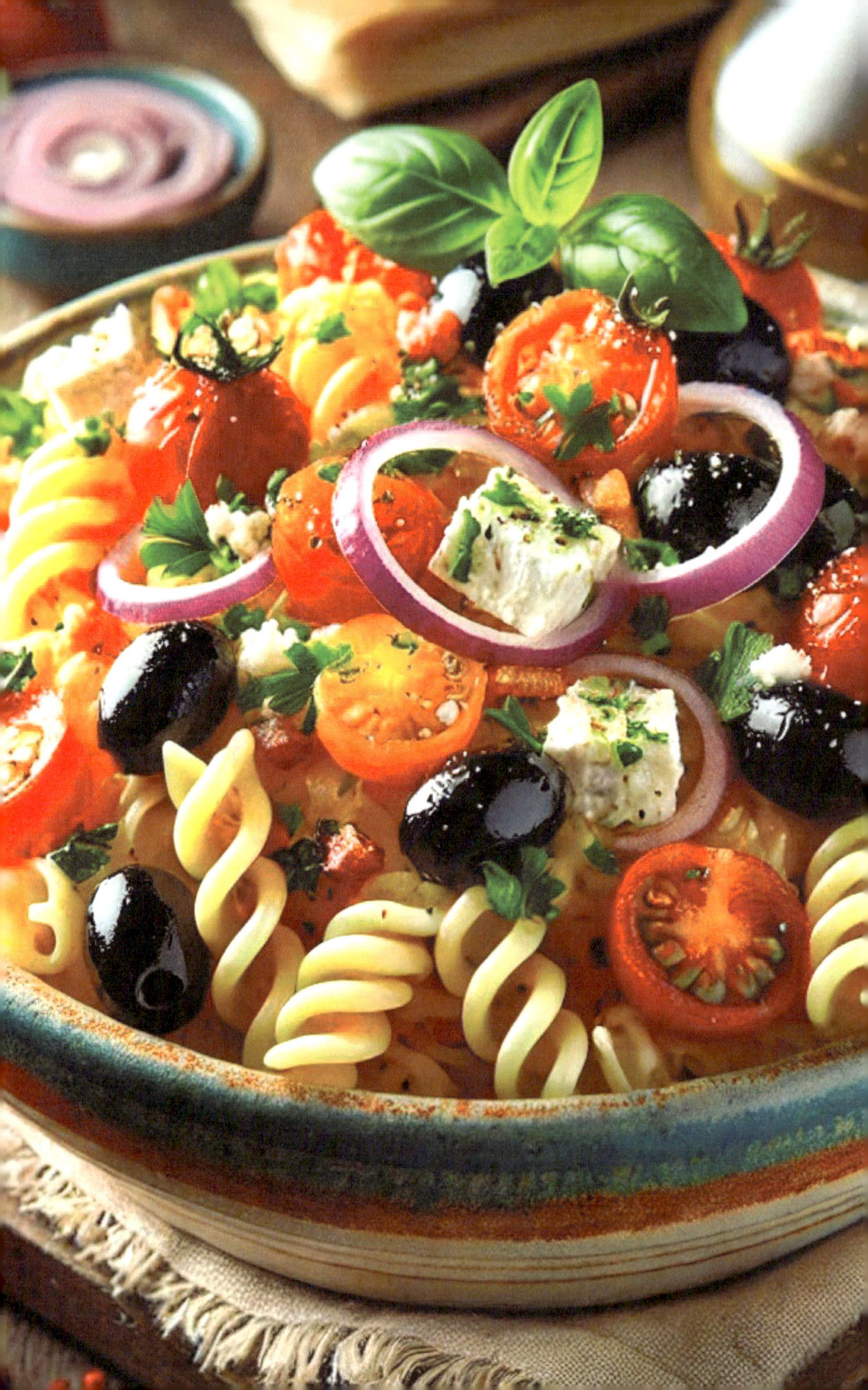

Mediterranean Pasta Dish

This simple dish has an unexpected twist of flavor with the addition of cinnamon. Penne pasta holds up against the ground beef, but any other shaped noodle will work. You can also make this with ground turkey or even lamb.

Ingredients:
1 ½ pounds ground beef
1 medium onion (chopped)
1 15-ounce can of tomato sauce
2 ½ cups uncooked penne pasta
2 garlic gloves (minced)
½ teaspoon salt
½ teaspoon ground cinnamon
½ cup (or more if desired) Parmesan cheese

Tools You'll Need:
Large skillet
Large pot
Measuring cups and spoons
Colander

Step-by-Step Instructions:

1 Make your sauce.
   In a large skillet, cook beef and onion over medium heat 8 to 10 minutes, or until beef is no longer pink. Drain excess liquid from meat. Add garlic and cook an additional two minutes. Stir in tomato sauce, salt, and cinnamon.

2 Cook pasta
   Fill a large pot with salted water and cook penne according to package directions. Drain.

3 Combine ingredients and serve.
   Spoon pasta into individual bowls and top with sauce and shredded Parmesan.

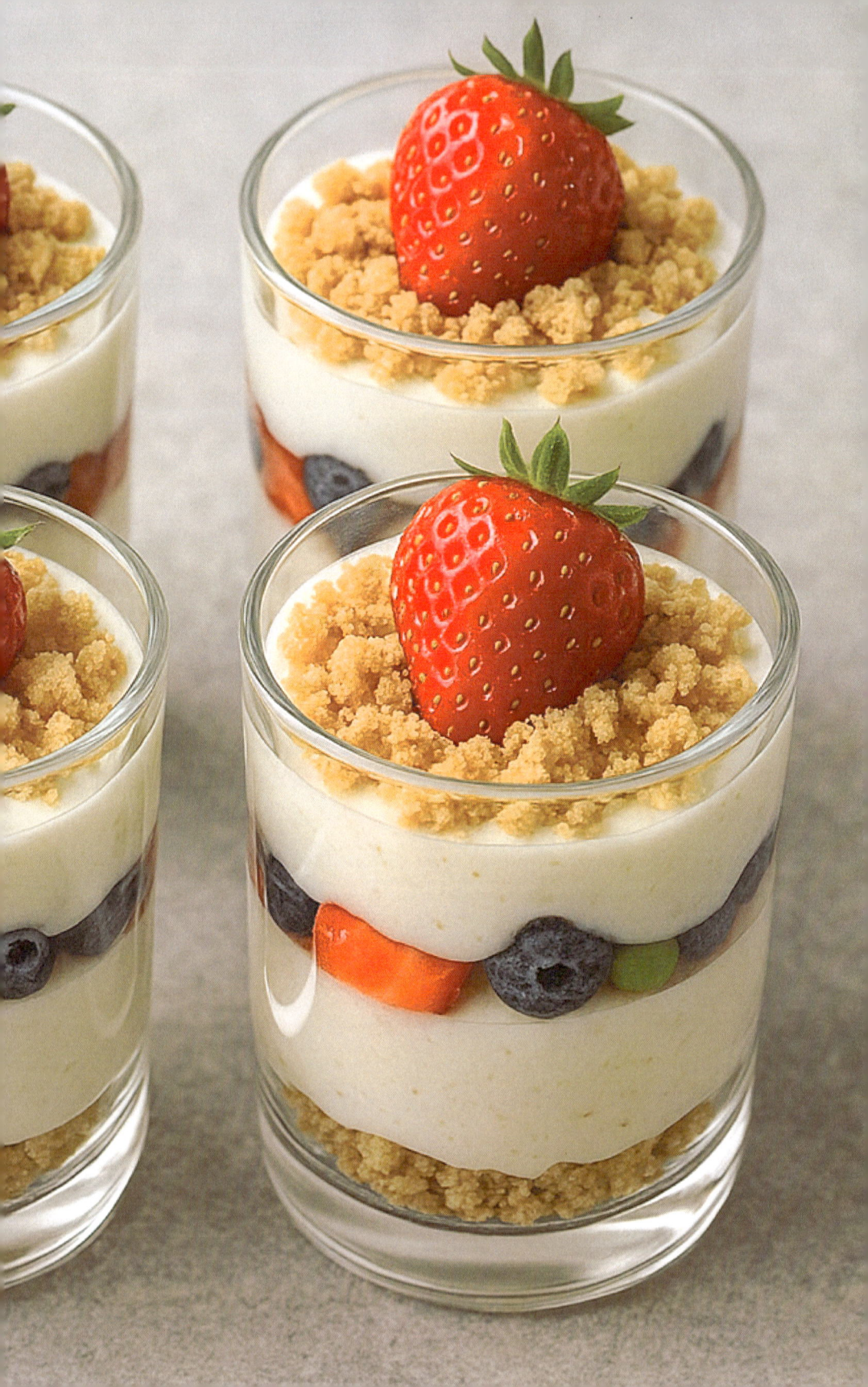

Mini French Yogurt Parfaits

Inspired by the light sweetness of French yogurt cakes and café-style fruit desserts—layered, soft, and no baking needed. You can use whatever ingredients you have on hand like fresh berries, jam, or even chocolate sauce. Be creative, and pretend you're at a sidewalk café in Paris while you eat them.

Ingredients:
Makes 4 small cups
1 cup plain or vanilla yogurt (Greek or regular)
2 tablespoons honey or fruit jam (strawberry, raspberry, or apricot)
½ teaspoon vanilla extract (optional)
½ cup soft fruit (like berries or banana slices)
4 crushed butter cookies (like Petit Beurre, shortbread, or graham crackers)

Step-by-Step Instructions:

1 **Prepare the yogurt mixture.**
In a bowl, mix yogurt with honey (or jam) and vanilla. Stir gently with a spoon until smooth and slightly sweet.

2 **Layer the dessert.**
In each cup:
> Add a spoon of crushed cookies
> Add a spoon of the yogurt mix
> Add some fruit
> Repeat the layers one more time

3 Top it off.
Sprinkle a little more cookie on top. Add a small piece of fruit as decoration if you like!

4 Chill or eat.
You can eat it right away, or chill in the fridge for 10–15 minutes to make it cold and creamy.

Tools You'll Need:
Spoon
Small bowl
4 clear cups or dessert bowls
Measuring spoons

Tips for Accessibility:
No oven or stove—just layering and stirring.

Cookie crumbs can be crushed in a plastic bag using hands.

Use pre-cut or soft fruits like banana slices or canned peaches.

Color-coded bowls for each ingredient can make it easier to follow steps.

Clear cups let you see your success layer by layer—a great visual reward!

Mongolian Breakfast Wraps

A warm flatbread filled with egg, cheese, and tender beef seasoned with Mongolian spices like ginger, garlic, and soy sauce. Try marinating your beef for an hour to really get the flavors to meld together. Mongolia is a desolate country, and they rely on spices to keep their meats tender in unforgiving weather. Chances are, you don't have to deal with the same conditions where you live, but when you eat these wraps you can pretend you are a hunter living in the frozen tundra.

Ingredients:

Makes 2 wraps
2 soft flatbreads (like tortillas or lavash – store-bought is okay!)
2 eggs
½ cup cooked ground beef (or shredded leftover beef – Mongolian style uses seasoned meat)
½ cup shredded cheese
1 tbsp soy sauce
1 tsp oil or butter
A pinch of black pepper

Optional Add-ins:
Chopped green onions
A few cucumber slices or shredded cabbage for crunch
Ketchup or plain yogurt on the side

Tools You'll Need:
Frying pan
Spatula
Small bowl
Spoon or fork
Plate

Tips for Accessibility:
Pre-cook the beef the night before or use leftover meat.

Everything can be done with one pan.

Wrapping the flatbread can be done by folding the bottom up, then the sides in.

Step-by-Step Instructions:

1 Warm the pan.
   Put your pan on medium heat and add a little oil or butter.

2 Cook the eggs.
   Crack both eggs into a bowl, beat them with a fork, and pour into the hot pan. Stir gently until scrambled and cooked through (about 2 minutes). Set eggs aside on a plate.

3 Heat the beef.
   In the same pan, add the cooked beef and pour in soy sauce. Stir for 1 minute to warm it up and add flavor. Sprinkle a little pepper.

4 Assemble the wrap.
   Place flatbreads on a plate. Add half the eggs, half the beef, and some cheese to each

one. Add green onions or veggies if you like.

5 **Wrap and toast.**
Fold like a burrito or roll it up. If you want it warm and toasty, place it back in the pan for 1 minute on each side until the cheese melts a bit.

6 **Eat and smile.**
Serve with ketchup or yogurt on the side. Eat with your hands or cut in half with a butter knife!

Tips for Accessibility:
Pre-cook the beef the night before or use leftover meat.
Everything can be done with one pan.
Wrapping the flatbread can be done by folding the bottom up, then the sides in.

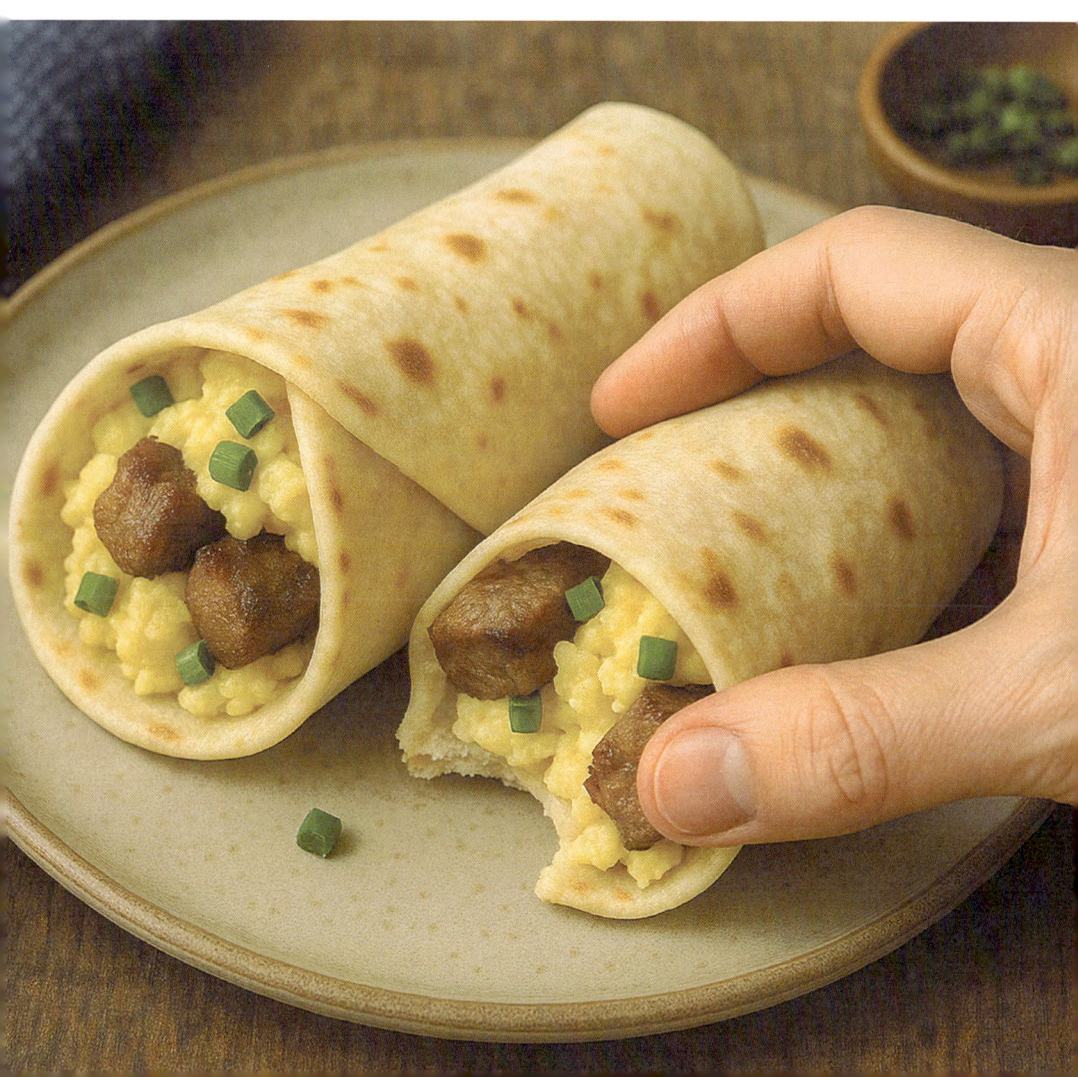

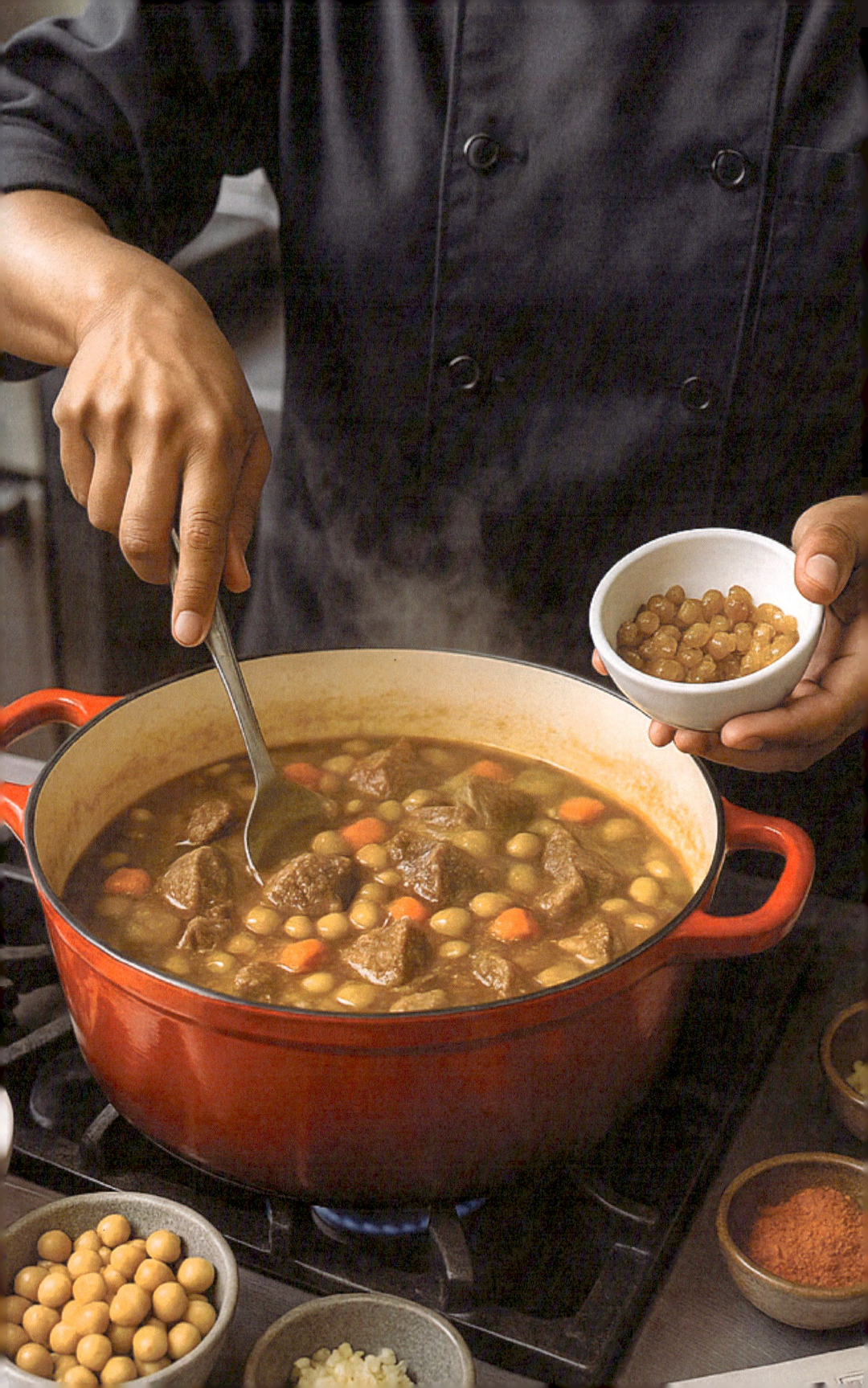

Moroccan Lamb Crockpot Stew

The slow cooking of a crockpot is ideal for lamb. And it's also a great way to meal prep and have something delicious waiting for you when you walk through the door after a long day. Lamb shanks are a very fatty meat so make sure to remove the excess fat before putting it in your crockpot so the stew doesn't become too oily. If you can use homemade chicken stock for this recipe it will really elevate the flavors, but boxed is fine too. Serve it with couscous or rice for a hearty and satisfying meal.

Ingredients:

2 small boneless lamb shanks with excess fat removed (5 to 6 pounds total)
3 cups chopped onion (about two large onions)
2 tablespoons olive oil
1 ½ teaspoons chili powder
1 ½ teaspoons ground turmeric
1 ½ teaspoons ground cumin
1 ½ teaspoons ground cardamom
3 garlic cloves, thinly sliced
1 tablespoon grated fresh ginger
1 4-inch cinnamon stick
1 28-ounce can diced tomatoes
1 pound russet or Yukon potatoes (peeled and diced into 1-inch pieces)
1 pound butternut squash (peeled and diced into 1-inch pieces

½ pound sweet potatoes (peeled and diced into 1-inch pieces)
½ cup diced apricots
2 cups chicken stock
2 tablespoons light brown sugar, lightly packed
4 lime slices
Salt and freshly ground pepper to taste

Tools You'll Need:

Medium bow
Wooden spoon or spatula
Knife
Measuring cups and spoons
Large skillet
Crockpot

Step-by-Step Instructions:

1 Prepare lamb for crockpot.
   Combine chili powder, turmeric, cumin, and cardamom in a bowl and then coat lamb with the spice mixture, making sure to cover on all sides. Heat oil on medium heat in a large skillet and sauté lamb on all sides. Stir in onion, garlic, and ginger and cook for an additional few minutes until onion is tender and translucent, then transfer lamb, onion, garlic, and ginger to crockpot.

2 Add the rest of ingredients to crock pot and stir to combine.
   Cook for three hours on low, raising lid to skim off fat ever so often.

3 Serve with rice or couscous.

Nana's Italian Roulade

This is another family recipe that is always a hit and helps me live my fantasies of traveling to Italy. A "roulade" is essentially a filled roll, and this one features juicy flank steak, Italian spices, and crisp bacon. It's also a nice addition to leftover spaghetti noodles that you may have in the fridge. You don't have to serve it over spaghetti, you can also serve it next to a salad, rice, or even gnocchi.

Ingredients:

4 bacon strips
1 beef flank steak (1 ½ to 2 pounds)
3 hard-boiled eggs, sliced thin
2 24-ounce jars of meatless pasta sauce
3 to 6 cups cooked spaghetti
2 garlic cloves (minced)
¾ teaspoon Italian seasoning
½ teaspoon salt
½ teaspoon pepper
¼ cup grated Parmesan cheese
2 tablespoons olive oil
2-3 tablespoons fresh parsley (chopped)

Tools You'll Need:

Large frying pan
Spoon
Small bowl
Measuring cups and spoons
A meat mallet or rolling pin
Microwave-safe plate
Paper towels
Large ovens safe baking pan or dish
Kitchen string or twine

Step-by-Step Instructions:

Tips for Accessibility:

Sometimes placing a piece of plastic wrap over the steak will make it easier to thin with a mallet.

1 Preheat your oven to 350 degrees and cook your bacon.
Place bacon on a microwave-safe plate lined with paper towels and cover with a moist paper towel—microwave on high 3 to 4 minutes or until partially cooked but not crisp.

2 Make your garlic mixture and prepare the flank steak.
In a small bowl, mix garlic, Italian seasoning, salt, and pepper. Spread your flank steak on a flat surface or cutting board and pound with a meat mallet or rolling pin until the steak is evenly thin enough to roll (roughly ¼ to ½ inch thick). Spread the garlic mixture over steak and sprinkle with Parmesan cheese. Layer with eggs and bacon to within one inch of the edges of the steak and sprinkle with parsley.

3 Roll your steak and lightly brown it on the stove.
Starting on the long side of the steak, roll up like a jelly roll along the grain into one large roll, then tie at 1 and 1/2 -inch intervals with kitchen string or twine. Heat olive oil in a large frying pan over medium-high heat until browned on all sides. Transfer to oven dish and cover with pasta sauce.

4 **Bake, cool, and slice your roulade.**
Bake roulade for 1 to 1 ½ hours until meat is tender. Remove from the dish and let cool for five minutes before removing the string and cutting into slices. Serve with sauce over spaghetti and sprinkle with additional Parmesan if desired.

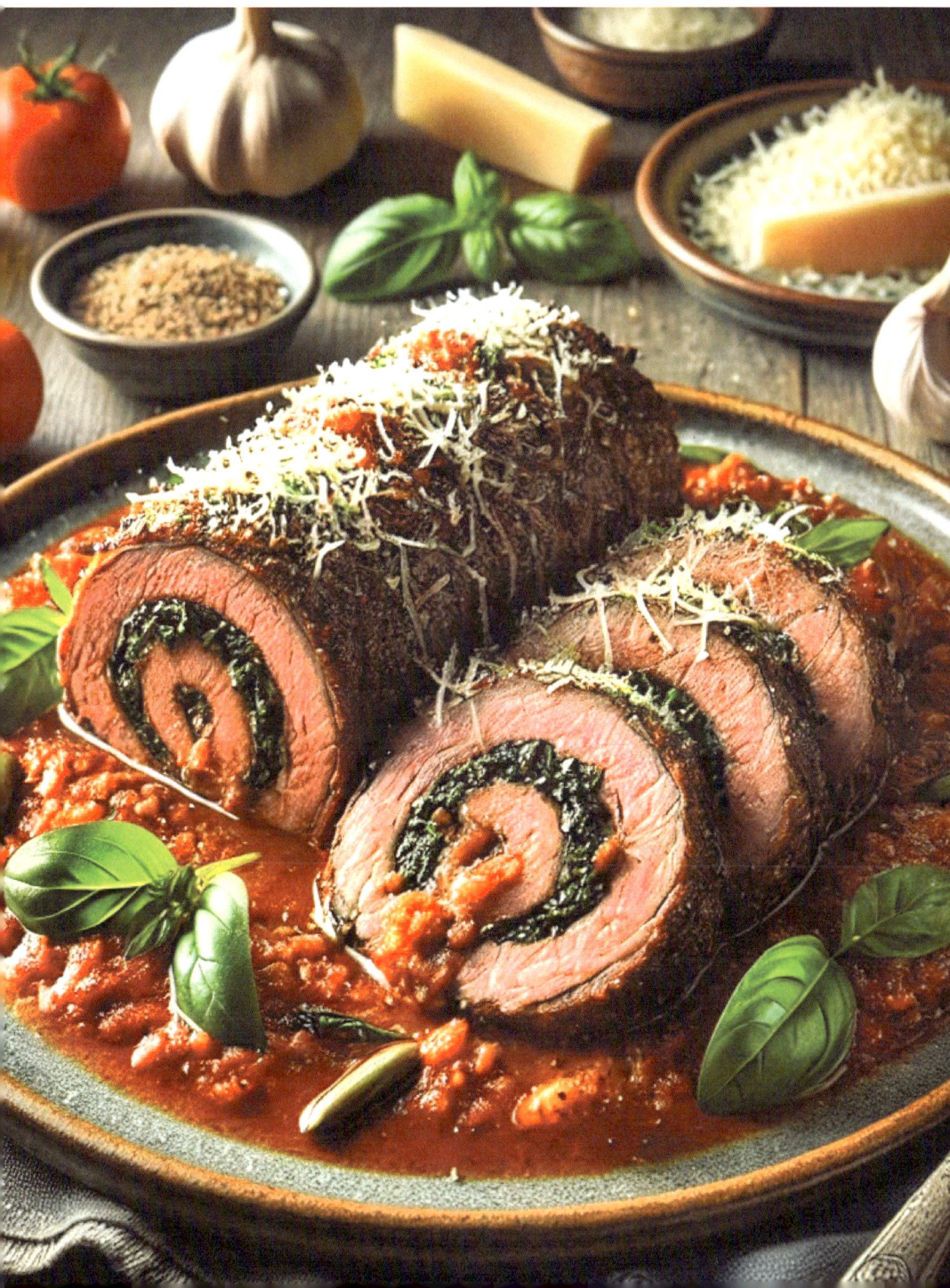

Norwegian Apple Cream Cups

A simple, sweet dessert with warm cinnamon apples and creamy vanilla yogurt—like a soft apple pie in a cup. Topping them with crushed oat cookies or granola is well worth it for the crunch and added texture.

Ingredients:

2 apples (or use 1 cup canned apples or pre-cut slices)
1 tablespoon butter or margarine
1 tablespoon brown sugar
½ teaspoon cinnamon
1 cup plain or vanilla yogurt (or vanilla pudding)
Optional: crushed oat cookies or granola for topping

Tools You'll Need:

Small frying pan or micro-wave-safe bowl
Spoon
Measuring spoons
4 small cups or bowls

Step-by-Step Instructions:

1 Cook the Apples

Peel and chop apples into small pieces (get help if needed).

Stovetop: Cook apples with butter, sugar, and cinnamon in a small pan for 5–7 minutes until soft.

Microwave: Place everything in a bowl, cover, and heat for 3 minutes, stirring halfway.

2 Cool the Apples

Let the cooked apples cool for a few minutes so they don't melt the yogurt.

3 Make the Cups

In each cup, add a spoon of yogurt. Then add a spoon of apples. Repeat for two layers.

4 Add Topping (Optional)

Sprinkle crushed cookies or granola on top for crunch.

5 Chill or Eat

You can eat it warm or refrigerate for 10 minutes to serve cold.

Tips for Accessibility:

Use canned or pre-sliced apples to skip chopping.

Yogurt is easy to scoop and layer.

All ingredients are soft and easy to eat with a spoon.

Microwave option avoids stovetop if needed.

Topping step can be a fun sensory moment—crunch and sprinkle!

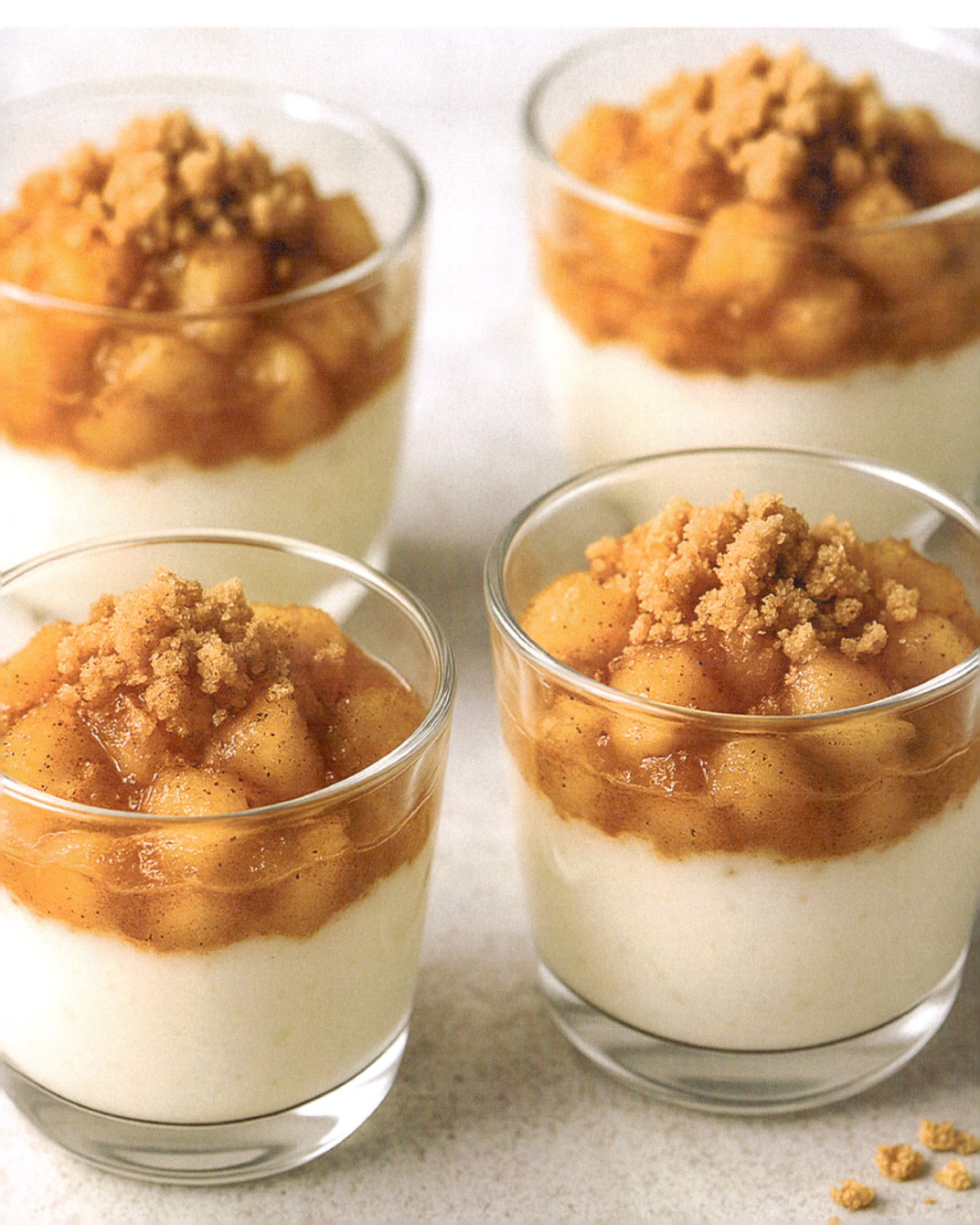

Norwegian Fish & Potato Boats

Soft baked potato halves filled with creamy fish and dill—warm, comforting, and easy to eat. In Norway, fish is a staple food, and these potato boats feature typical Scandinavian flavors of dill and cream. This dish is a special treat on cold evenings.

Ingredients:
Makes 4 potato boats – 2 servings
2 large potatoes (russet or baking potatoes)
1 small can of tuna or cooked white fish (like halibut)
3 tablespoons plain yogurt or sour cream
¼ teaspoon dried dill (or fresh, if available)
Salt and pepper to taste
2 tablespoons shredded cheese (optional)
1 teaspoon butter or oil

Tools You'll Need:
Microwave or oven
Spoon
Small bowl
Fork
Baking tray or micro-wave-safe plate

Step-by-Step Instructions:

1 Cook the Potatoes

Wash the potatoes. Poke a few holes in each with a fork.

Microwave: Place on a plate and microwave for 8–10 minutes (flip halfway) until soft.

Oven: Bake at 200°C (400°F) for 45–60 minutes until soft.

2 Make the Filling

In a bowl, mix the fish, yogurt or sour cream, dill, salt, and pepper with a spoon until creamy.

3 Scoop and Stuff

Let the potatoes cool slightly. Cut in half lengthwise. Use a spoon to scoop out some of the inside into the bowl with the fish mixture. Mash and mix everything together.

4 Fill the Boats

Spoon the creamy fish filling back into the potato skins. Sprinkle cheese on top if using.

5 Heat and Serve

Microwave: Heat the stuffed potatoes for 1–2 more minutes to warm and melt the cheese.

Oven: Bake for 10 minutes until golden and hot.

6 Eat and Enjoy
  Serve warm with a spoon or fork. Soft, scoopable, and full of cozy Norwegian flavor!

Tips for Accessibility:

Use canned tuna to avoid cooking raw fish.
Microwave option reduces cooking time and simplifies steps.
Yogurt and fish can be mixed with a spoon—no knives needed.
Potatoes act as edible bowls—no extra plates required!

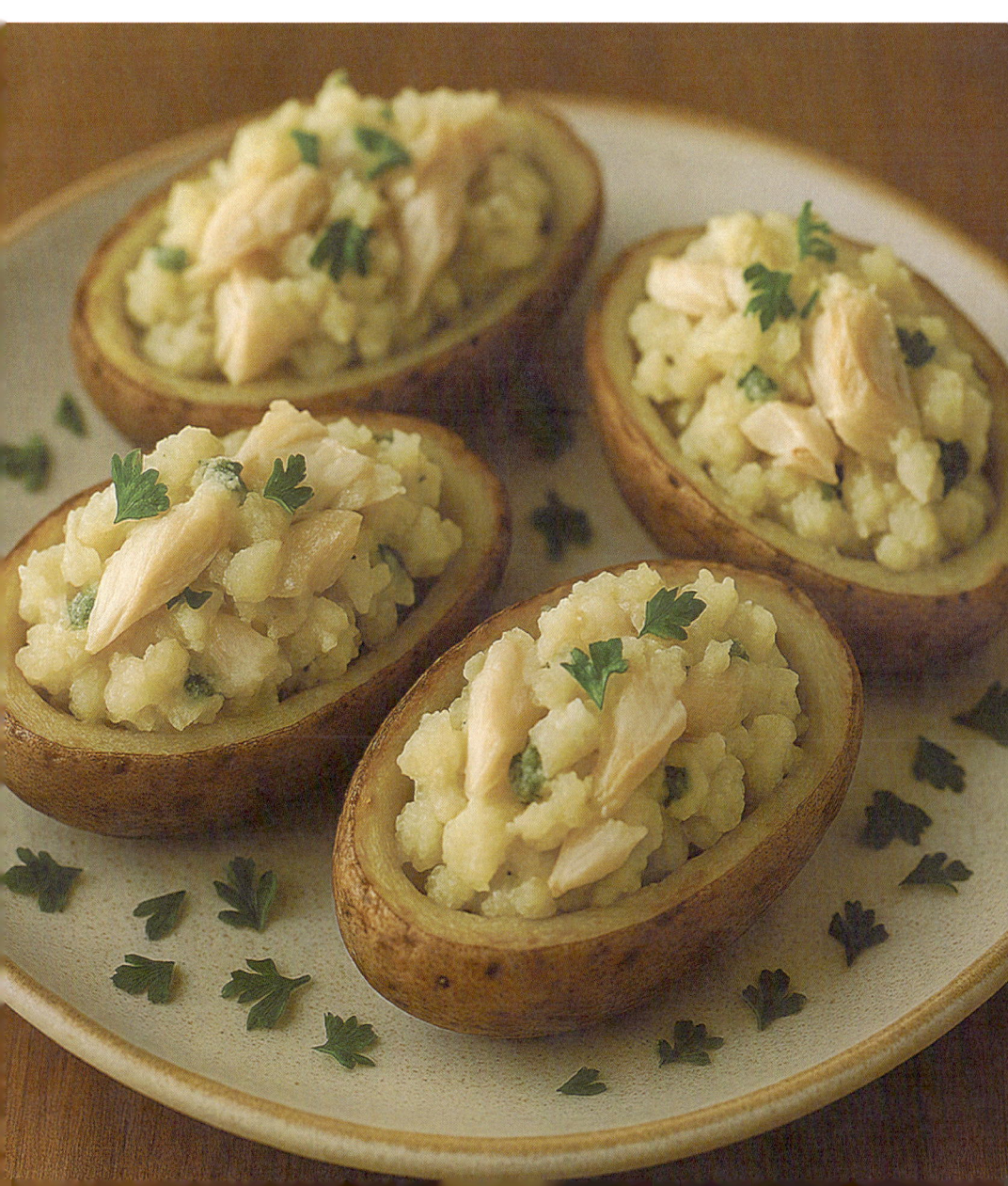

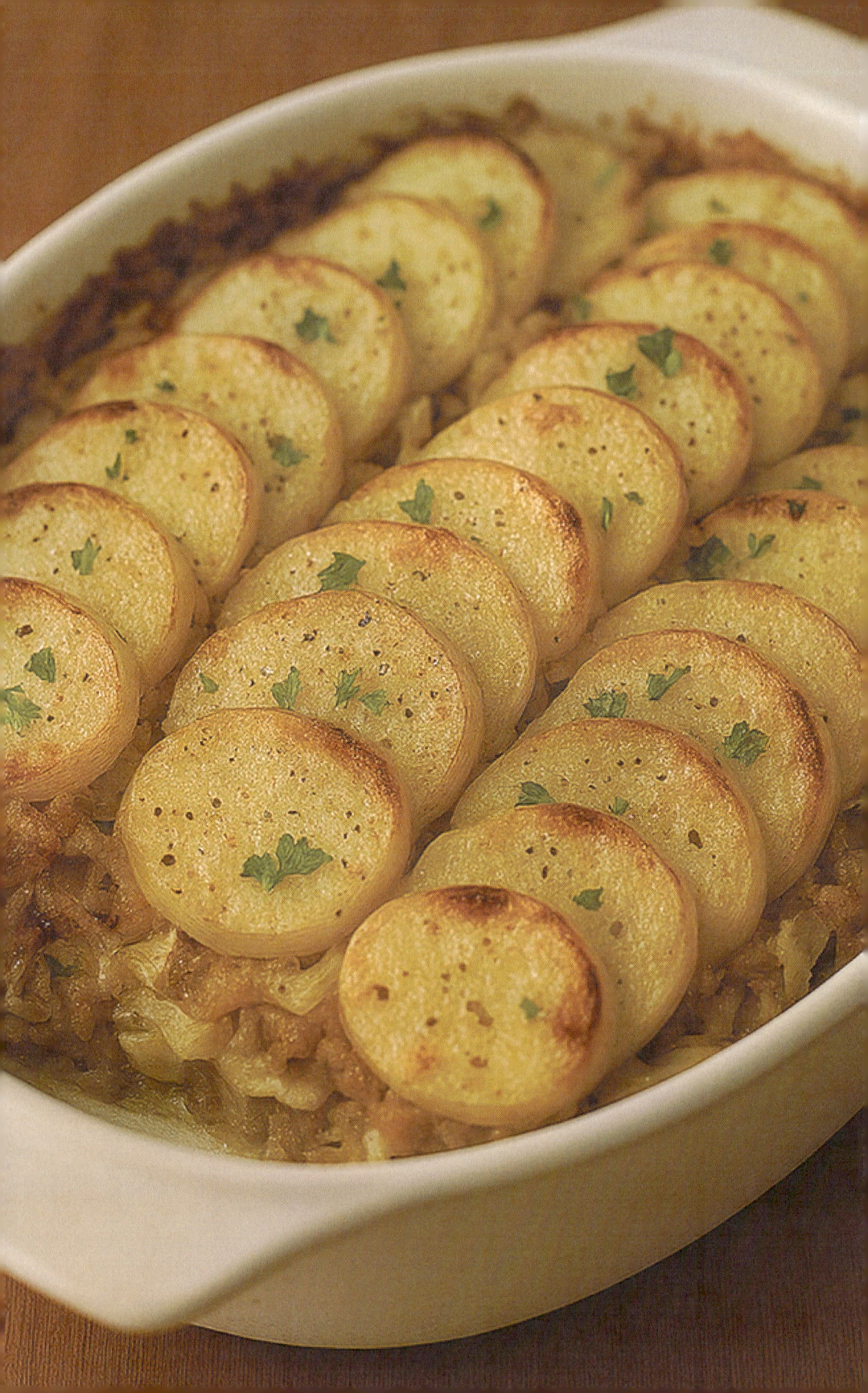

Polish Pierogi-Style Potato & Cabbage Bake

A cozy, soft, one-dish dinner with mashed potatoes, sautéed cabbage, cheese, and gentle seasoning—tastes like pierogi in a bowl. Pierogies are a popular, dumpling-like dish popular throughout Europe but especially in Poland.

Ingredients:

Makes 3–4 servings

2 cups mashed potatoes (pre-made, instant, or fresh)

1 cup cooked cabbage or sauerkraut (mild, drained)

½ cup shredded cheese (cheddar or farmer's cheese)

1 tablespoon butter or oil

½ teaspoon onion powder

Salt and pepper to taste

Optional: a dollop of sour cream on top

Tools You'll Need:

Medium mixing bowl

Spoon

Baking dish (8x8 or similar)

Oven or toaster oven

Tips for Accessibility:

Use instant mashed potatoes or refrigerated pre-made mash.

Use bagged sauerkraut or cooked cabbage (jarred or canned is fine).

Onion powder gives flavor without chopping.

Spoon mixing and baking keep it safe and tactile.

It's soft, warm, and easy to scoop—ideal for comfort and confidence.

Step-by-Step Instructions:

1 **Preheat oven.**
Set oven or toaster oven to 180°C (350°F).

2 **Mix the ingredients.**
In a mixing bowl, stir together mashed potatoes, cooked cabbage or sauerkraut, cheese, onion powder, and butter. Add salt and pepper to taste.

3 **Scoop into a dish.**
Spoon the mixture into a greased baking dish. Smooth the top with the back of a spoon.

4 **Bake until warm.**
Bake for 15–20 minutes until heated through and lightly golden on top.

5 **Serve and top with sour cream.**
Scoop onto a plate or into a bowl. Add a spoonful of sour cream if you like.

Russian Fish Au Gratin

"Au Gratin" is a French culinary method where something is topped with breadcrumbs or cheese (or both) and then browned, usually in the oven. It is more commonly seen with potatoes, but this Russian spin on au gratin is a great way to incorporate some seafood into the diets of people who otherwise don't like fish.

Ingredients:

3 pounds of fish fillets (Tilapia, Bass, or Catfish are good options), cut into strips
1 small potato (russet or Yukon Gold), peeled and sliced thin
1 cup sliced mushrooms (Cremini or button)
⅓ cup whole milk
½ cup heavy cream
2 eggs (yolks and whites separated)
1 ½ cups grated mozzarella cheese
1 tablespoon grated Parmesan cheese
½ onion sliced thin
3 tablespoons white flour
2 teaspoons vegetable oil
2 tablespoons butter
½ teaspoon dried parsley

Tools You'll Need:

Medium non-stick skillet
Three large plates
Measuring cups and spoons
Medium bowl
Small bowl
2 medium-sized baking dishes

½ teaspoon dried basil
½ teaspoon white pepper
½ teaspoon salt
1 tablespoon lemon juice
1 teaspoon salt
Optional: 1 teaspoon whiskey

Step-by-Step Instructions:

1 Marinate fish.

Dry fish fillet slices with paper towels and place on a plate. Add lemon juice, rub with salt and black pepper, and marinate in the fridge for 20 to 30 minutes.

2 Cook your mushrooms and onions.

Heat a teaspoon of oil in a non-stick skillet and once hot, add mushrooms and stir-fry until they turn soft. Add salt, pepper (and whiskey if using), and continue to stir-fry until all the liquid evaporates and mushrooms turn golden. Put mushrooms on a plate and set aside. Heat the rest of your oil in the same skillet and add the onion, stir-frying until the onions turn soft and golden. Put on the same plate and set aside.

3 Preheat your oven to 350 degrees and prepare your au gratin mixture.

Add your heavy cream and milk into a medium-sized bowl, add parsley, basil, white pepper, salt, and egg yolks, and whisk with a fork. Place your flour on a big plate and your egg whites into a small bowl.

4 **Coat your fish and fry it.**

Heat 1 tablespoon butter in a non-stick skillet on medium high heat. Coat each side of fish fillet with flour and dip both sides of fillet in egg whites and place in the skillet immediately. Fry fish until the bottom side turns golden, the flip to fry the other side. When both sides are done, remove from heat and set on a plate.

5 **Prepare and bake your fish.**

Grease two medium-sized baking dish with the rest of the butter. Place half the onion in both dishes, add fish on top and place potato slices against the walls of each dish. Add the rest of your onion on top of each fish, then top with mushrooms. Fill each dish with the au gratin milk mixture, filling to about 1-inch of the top of each dish. Top with a thin layer of Mozzarella cheese, then sprinkle with Parmesan cheese. Cook for 25 minutes until top is golden and cheese is bubbly. Let cook and then slice into squares to serve.

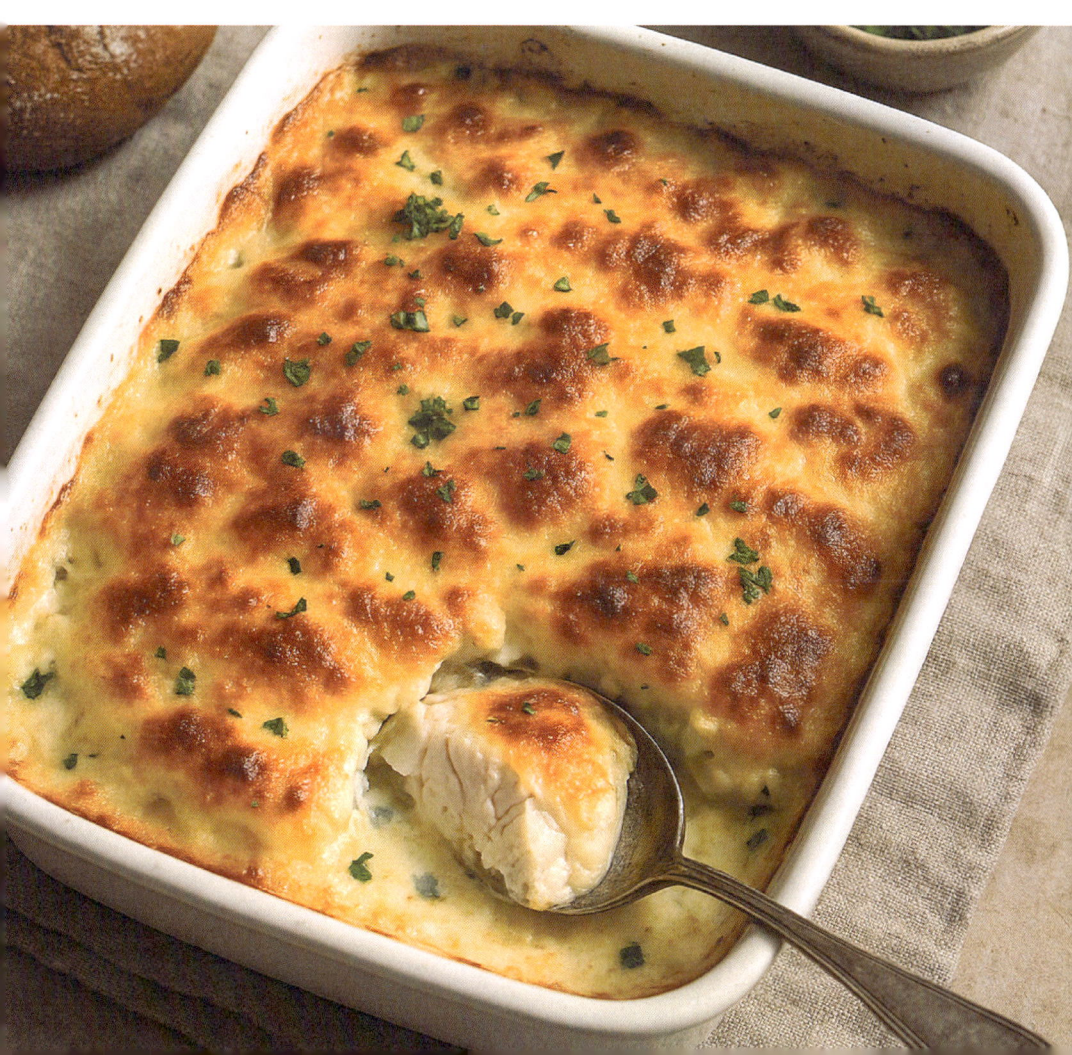

Sweet Yam Breakfast Boats

Inspired by the Nigerian love for yams and eggs, these oven-baked yam "boats" are filled with creamy eggs. You don't have to use Nigerian yams (also known as Cassava), but if you can find them at the specialty section of the grocery store you'll find them to be very sweet and great for baking. Cassava flour is a popular gluten free flour made from these Nigerian yams.

Ingredients:

Makes 2 servings

1 medium yam or sweet potato (Nigerian yams are best, but any sweet potato works!)

2 eggs

2 tablespoons evaporated milk or plain yogurt

A pinch of salt

A pinch of ground pepper (optional)

1 tablespoon vegetable oil or melted butter

Optional: 1 tablespoon grated cheese or cooked beans for topping

Tools You'll Need:

Oven or toaster oven

Spoon

Bowl

Fork

Baking dish or foil

Step-by-Step Instructions:

1 Bake the yam.

Wash the yam and poke a few holes in it with a fork.

Bake at 200°C (400°F) for 45–60 minutes, or microwave for 6–8 minutes until soft.

Let it cool slightly.

2 Make the egg mixture.

In a bowl, crack the eggs. Add milk (or yogurt), a pinch of salt, and pepper. Beat with a fork until smooth.

3 Prepare the boats.

Slice the baked yam in half lengthwise. Use a spoon to gently scoop out a little of the center to make space (like a shallow boat). Place yam halves in a small baking dish or on foil.

4 Fill and bake.

Pour the egg mixture into the hollowed yam halves. Add cheese or beans if you like. Bake again at 180°C (350°F) for 12–15 minutes, until the eggs are set.

5 Cool and serve.

Let it cool slightly before serving. Eat with a spoon or pick up and bite if it's firm!

Tips for Accessibility:

Use pre-baked or microwaved yam for safety and speed.

All mixing is done with a fork—no knives required.

Boats are fun and easy to eat with hands or a spoon.

Familiar, comforting ingredients keep it culturally rooted and accessible.

Great sensory experience—soft, warm, sweet, and savory!

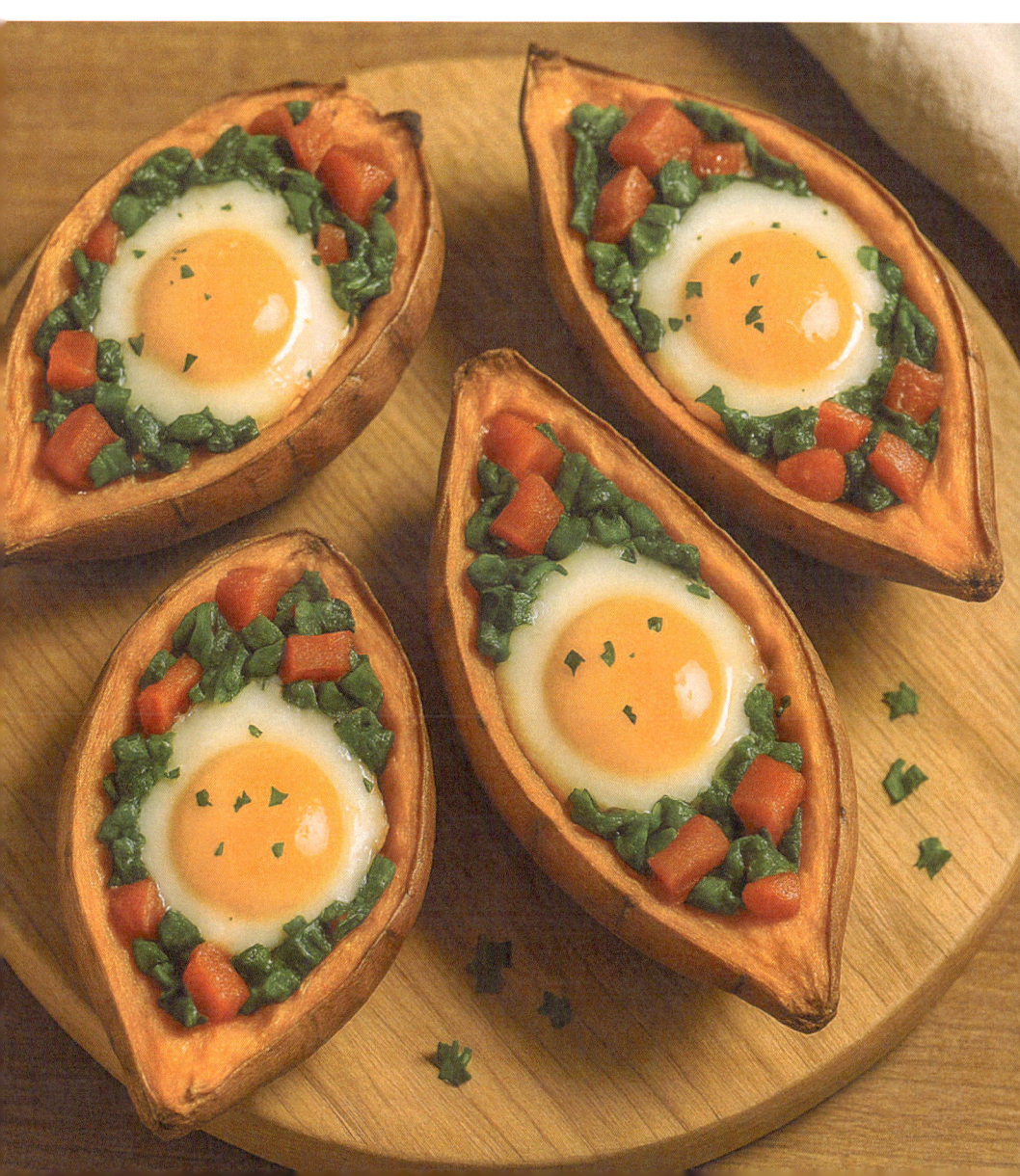

South African Bobotie Pie

This is a national dish in South Africa (pronounced Bo-bo-TIE) and is a real crowd pleaser as it makes enough to feed five to six people. You can make the pie a day before and chill in the fridge and make the topping before you are ready to put it in the oven.

Ingredients:
2 slices white bread
1 lb. lean minced beef (or ground turkey)
2 onions (chopped)
1 tbsp butter
2 garlic cloves
1 tsp. dried thyme herbs
1 tablespoon allspice
2 tablespoons peach or mango chutney
3 bay leaves

For the topping:
1 cup cream
2 eggs

Tools You'll Need:
Medium saucepan
Large ovenproof dish or baking pan
Measuring cups and spoons
Medium mixing bowl

Step-by-Step Instructions:

1 Heat oven to 350 degrees.

2 Soak your bread.
Place your bread into a medium bowl and pour cold water over it until it is fully submerged. Set it aside to soak.

3 Saute your onions and beef (or turkey).
Heat your butter in a medium skillet on medium heat and sauté your onions, stirring often, for 10 minutes or until soft and golden brown. Add the garlic and beef to the pan. Stir well, crushing the garlic until it changes color and the meat is fully cooked through. Add in the allspice, curry powder, thyme, chutney, and two of the bay leaves. Add 1 teaspoon salt and ground pepper. Cover and simmer for 10 minutes. Squeeze the excess water from the soaking bread and mix it into the meat mixture until well blended. Add the mixture to your oven-safe dish and smooth down the top (you can place this in the fridge overnight if you're not ready to cook it yet; otherwise, continue to the next steps.)

4 Make your topping.
Mix your cream and eggs with 1 teaspoon salt. Pour mixture over the meat and top with the remaining bay leaf.

5 Bake for 35-40 minutes.

Bake until the topping is set and starting to turn a golden brown. Remove from the oven and let sit for five minutes before cutting and serving. Enjoy!

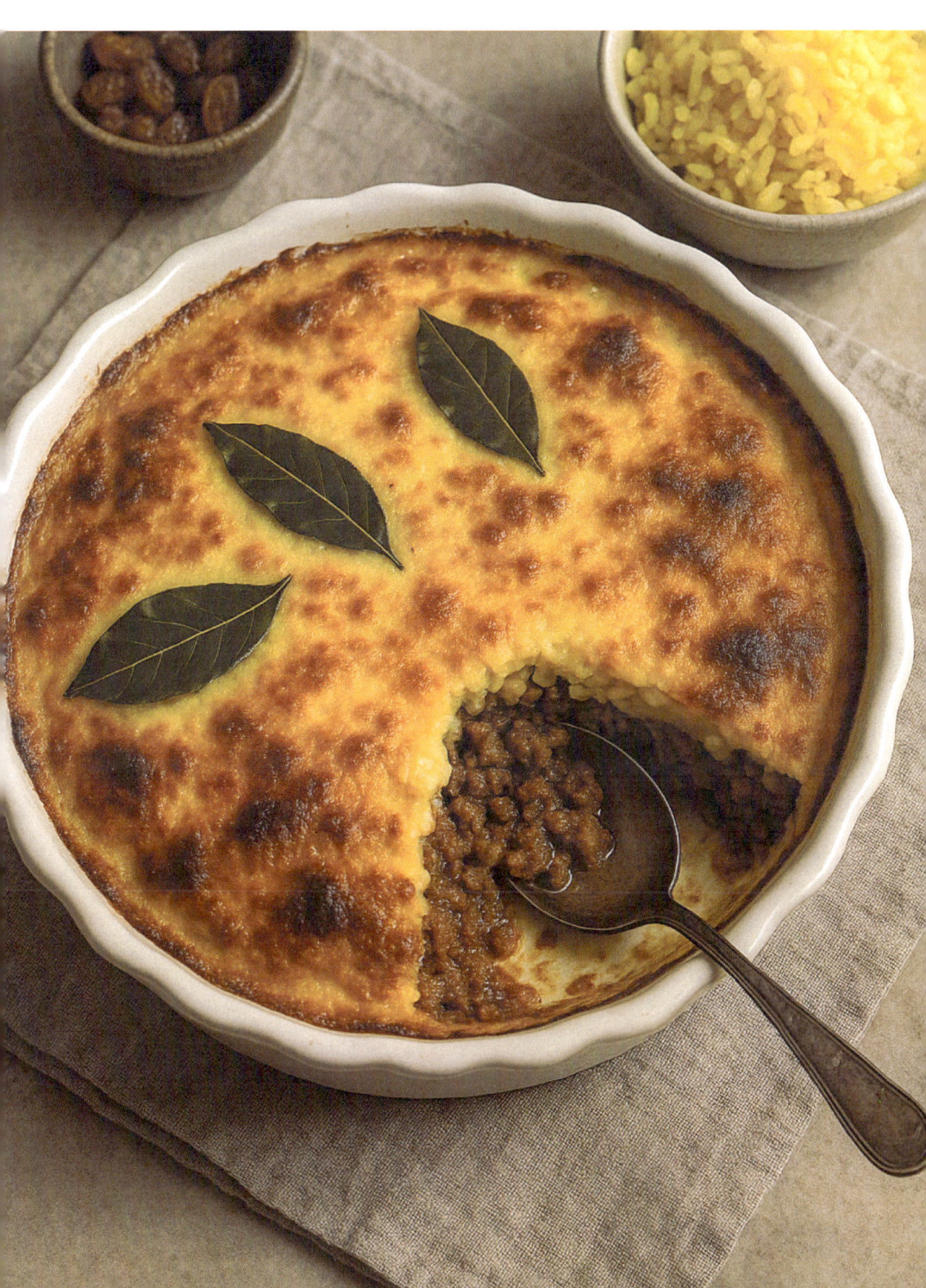

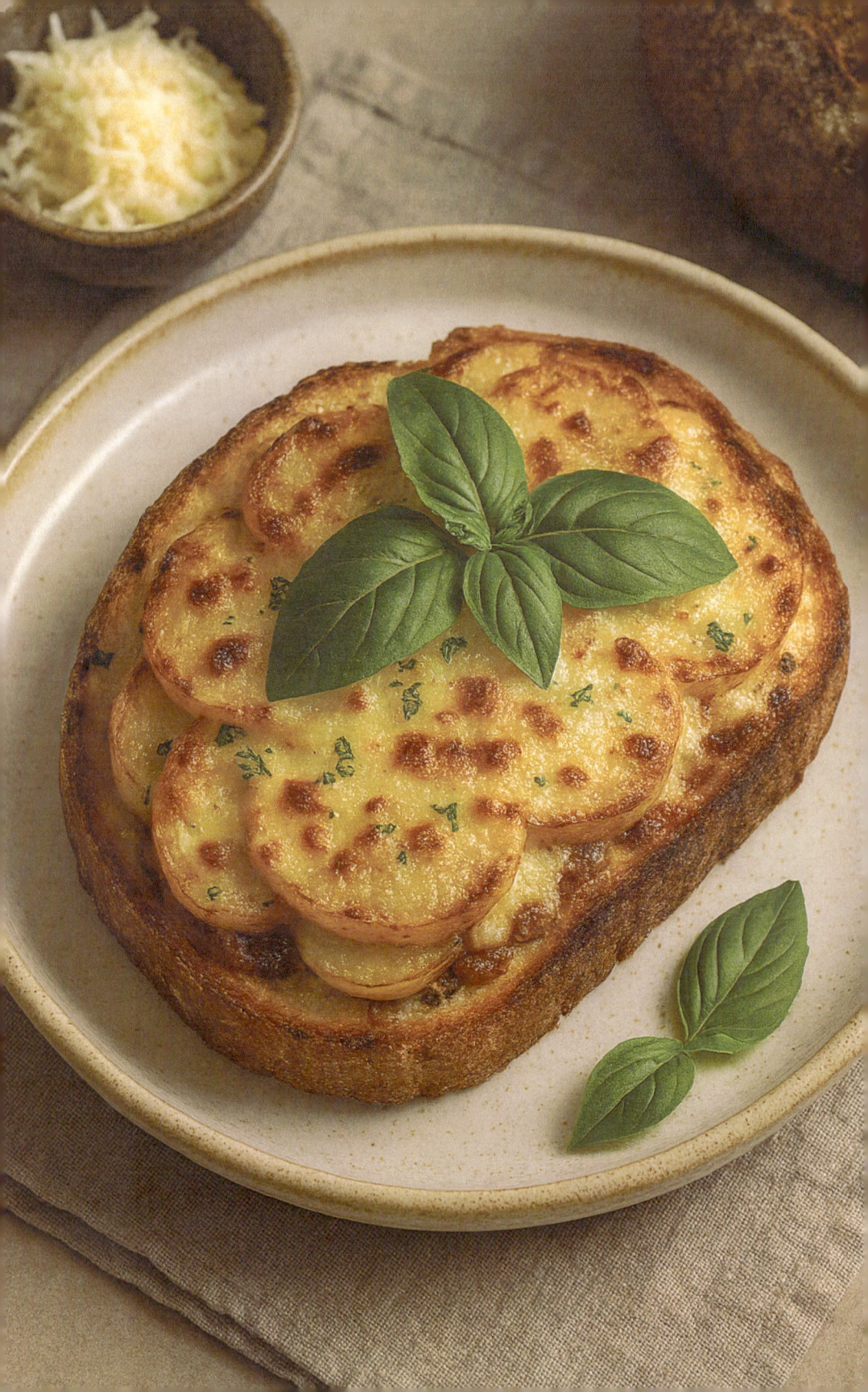

Spanish Potato Toast Melt

A warm, soft open-faced sandwich with mashed potatoes, tomatoes, and melted cheese—flavors of Spain with easy steps and no slicing. Manchego cheese is a more authentic cheese to use for this, but mozzarella will work as well. This is also a good use for that leftover crusty bread you might have and not know what to do with.

Ingredients:

Makes 2 melts

2 slices of bread (rustic, sandwich, or whatever you like)

½ cup instant mashed potatoes (or leftover mashed potatoes)

2 tablespoons canned diced tomatoes (drained) or tomato sauce

½ teaspoon olive oil (optional)

¼ teaspoon garlic powder

2 tablespoons shredded cheese (Manchego or mozzarella)

A pinch of salt and pepper

Tools You'll Need:

Bowl and spoon
Toaster oven or oven
Baking tray or foil
Plate

Tips for Accessibility:

Use instant mashed potatoes for simplicity.

Canned tomato requires no cutting or cooking.

Toasting everything together in one step keeps it safe and easy.

Soft, savory, and full of texture—ideal for sensory satisfaction.

No knives or stove needed—just stirring, spreading, and toasting.

Step-by-Step Instructions:

1 Make the Tomato Spread
In a bowl, mix the canned tomatoes (or sauce), olive oil, garlic powder, and a pinch of salt. Mash gently with a spoon.

2 Prepare the Bread Base
Toast the bread lightly so it holds the toppings better.

3 Layer the Toasts
Spread mashed potatoes on each piece of toast. Spoon the tomato mixture on top of the potatoes. Sprinkle cheese on top of everything.

4 Melt and Warm
Place the toasts on a baking tray. Bake or toast in the oven at 180°C (350°F) for about 8–10 minutes, until cheese melts.

5 Cool and Serve
Let cool slightly. Serve warm with a napkin or on a plate. Eat with hands or a fork!

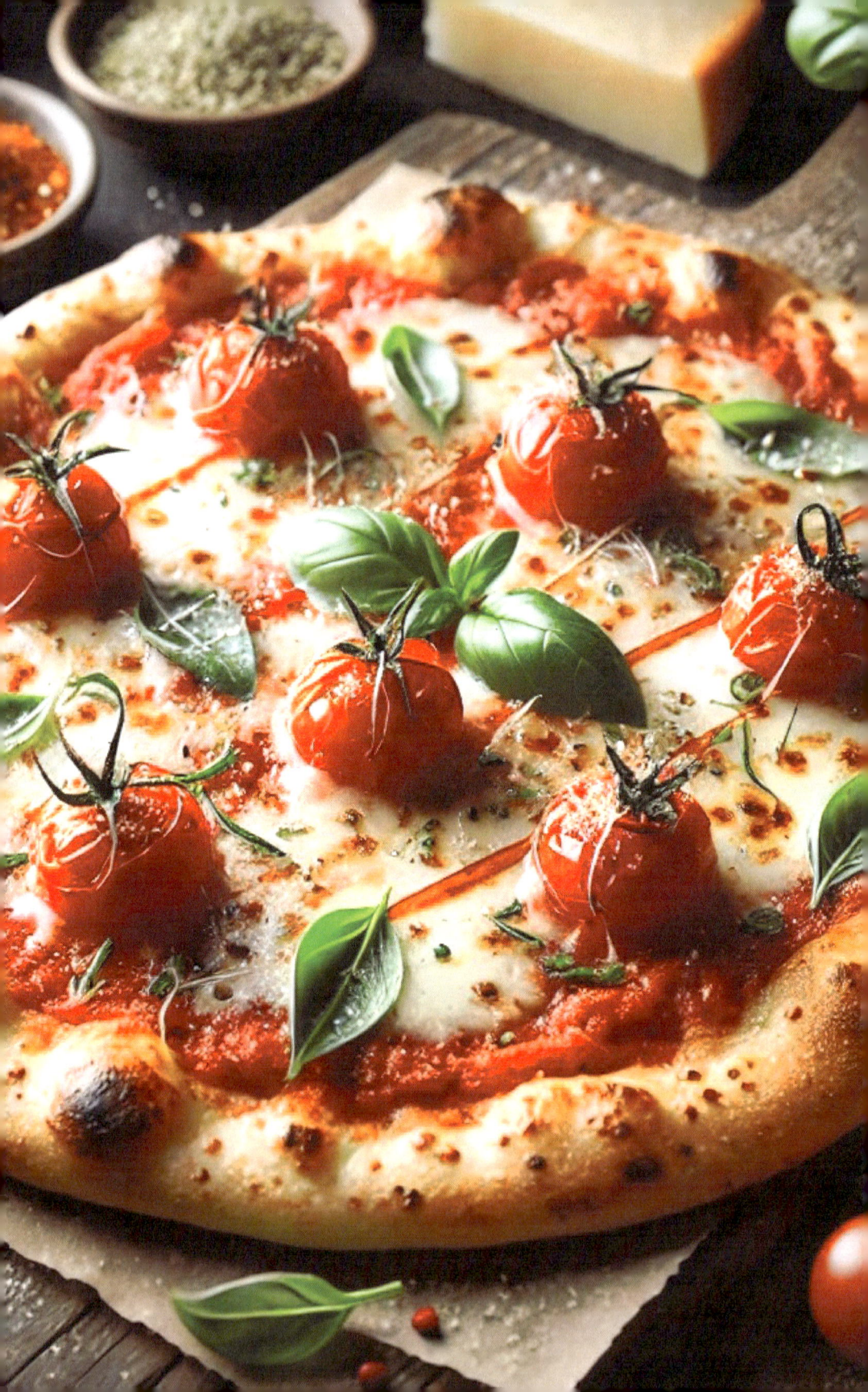

Spenser's Easy Pizza

You can have this pizza ready in less time than it takes to order one and have it delivered. Experiment with whatever toppings you like, and even try a different sauce like Alfredo for a white pizza. If you have a couple of flat bread crusts on hand, you can even have your friends assemble their pizzas and share your creations. I use my toaster oven for this, but if you don't have one just put the crust directly on the rack in your oven or on a pizza flat pan if you have one.

Ingredients:
1 Flatbread crust
½ jar of pizza sauce
2 cups mozzarella shredded cheese
12 slices of pepperoni
1 teaspoon garlic powder
Optional: sliced onion, black olives, bell pepper, basil, etc.

Tools You'll Need:
Optional: pizza pan
Measuring cups and spoons
Spatula or wooden spoon

Step-by-Step Instructions:

1 Heat your oven or toaster oven to 350 degrees.

2 Assemble your pizza.
   Spread on your pizza sauce using a spoon, then sprinkle on the mozzarella and add whichever toppings you like. Toast in the oven or toaster for roughly 10 minutes, or an additional 5 minutes if you like the crust a little darker. Remove carefully and let sit for a few minutes before slicing and serving.

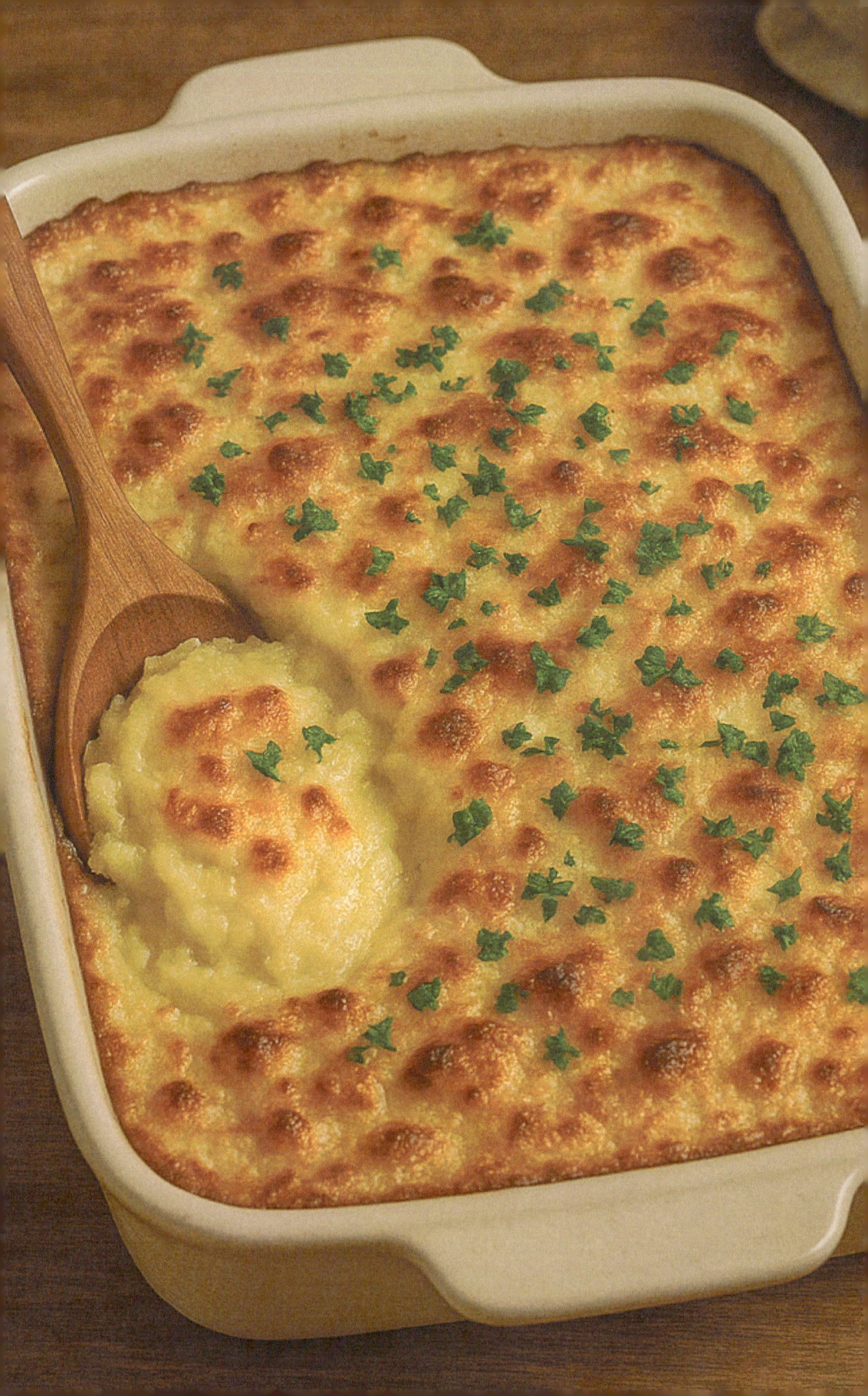

Ukrainian Cheesy Mashed Potato Bake

A warm, creamy potato-and-cheese casserole inspired by varenyky, which are Ukrainian dumplings filled with cheese and sometimes sweet fillings. They are traditionally served at festive gatherings and are considered a symbol of prosperity.

Ingredients:
Makes 2–3 servings
2 cups mashed potatoes (leftover, instant, or refrigerated)
½ cup cottage cheese or ricotta cheese
½ cup shredded cheese (mozzarella, cheddar, or a mix)
1 egg
½ teaspoon onion powder
A pinch of salt and pepper
Optional topping: a spoonful of sour cream and chopped dill or chives

Tools You'll Need:
Medium mixing bowl
Spoon
Baking dish (8x8 or any small oven-safe dish)
Oven or toaster oven

Tips for Accessibility:
No peeling or chopping—use instant mashed potatoes or leftovers.

Cottage cheese adds Ukrainian flavor without complicated prep.

Baking avoids stovetop risks and allows hands-free cooking time.

Spoon mixing and scooping are simple and safe steps.

Soft, comforting textures are easy to chew and enjoy.

Step-by-Step Instructions:

1 **Preheat the oven.**
Set your oven or toaster oven to 180°C (350°F).

2 **Mix the ingredients.**
In a bowl, combine mashed potatoes, cottage cheese, shredded cheese, egg, onion powder, salt, and pepper. Mix until smooth and blended.

3 **Scoop into dish.**
Spoon the mixture into a greased baking dish. Use the back of the spoon to smooth the top.

4 **Bake in the oven.**
Bake for 25–30 minutes until hot and slightly golden on top. Let cool for 5 minutes before serving.

5 **Top and serve.**
Add a spoonful of sour cream on each serving. Sprinkle with fresh or dried dill if you like. Serve warm with a spoon or fork.

Zambian Nshima Veggie Bowls

This soft maize porridge is known in Zambia as nshima and is served with a colorful, tender tomato-spinach relish. The relish or topping on nshima is super important as this porridge tastes rather bland on its own.

Ingredients:
Makes 2 servings
For the nshima (thick corn porridge):
½ cup finely ground maize meal (or white cornmeal)
1½ cups water
A pinch of salt

For the veggie relish:
½ cup canned chopped tomatoes (with juice)
½ cup frozen chopped spinach (or cooked fresh)
1 tablespoon oil or butter
½ teaspoon onion powder
Salt to taste

Tools You'll Need:
Medium pot or saucepan
Spoon (for stirring and serving)
Serving bowls

Step-by-Step Instructions:

1 Make the nshima.
  In a pot, boil 1 cup of the water.
  In a separate cup, mix the maize meal with the remaining ½ cup of cold water.
  Slowly pour the maize mixture into the boiling water while stirring.
  Stir constantly for 5–7 minutes until thick, smooth, and doughy. Add a pinch of salt.
  Cover and let rest for a minute. Turn off the heat.

2 Make the veggie relish.
  In another pot or pan, heat oil and add tomatoes, spinach, onion powder, and a pinch of salt.
  Stir and cook for 5–7 minutes until soft and combined. Turn off heat.

3 Assemble the bowl.
  Scoop a ball of nshima into each bowl (can use an ice cream scoop or spoon).
  Spoon veggie relish on the side or over the top.

4 Eat and enjoy.
  Everything is soft, warm, and can be eaten with a spoon or your hands if preferred!

Tips for Accessibility:

Nshima uses repetitive stirring—great for sensory feedback.

No chopping required—use canned and frozen ingredients.

Soft texture means easy chewing and swallowing.

Mixing and scooping steps are safe and satisfying.

Simple seasoning lets the person taste and adjust on their own.

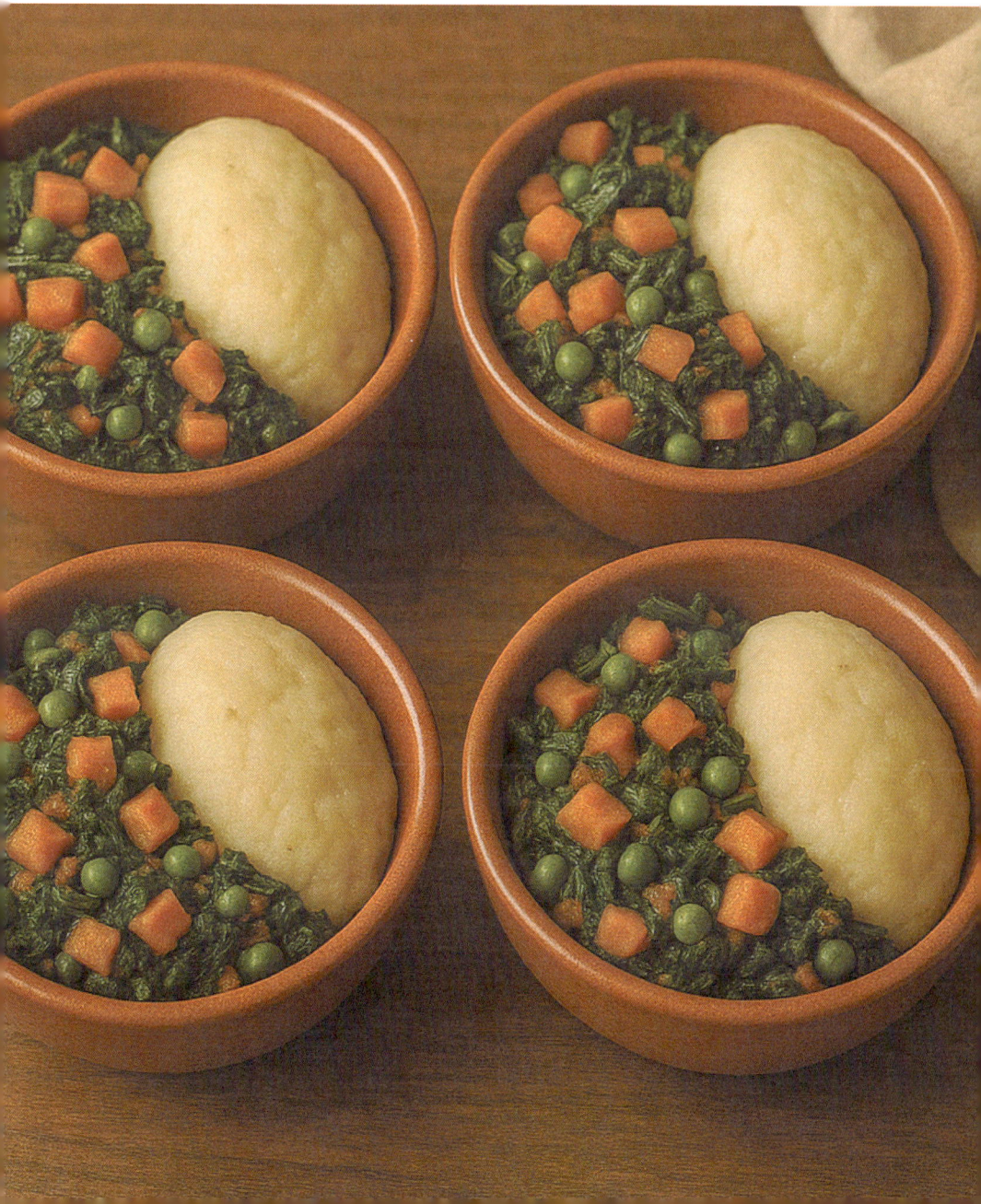

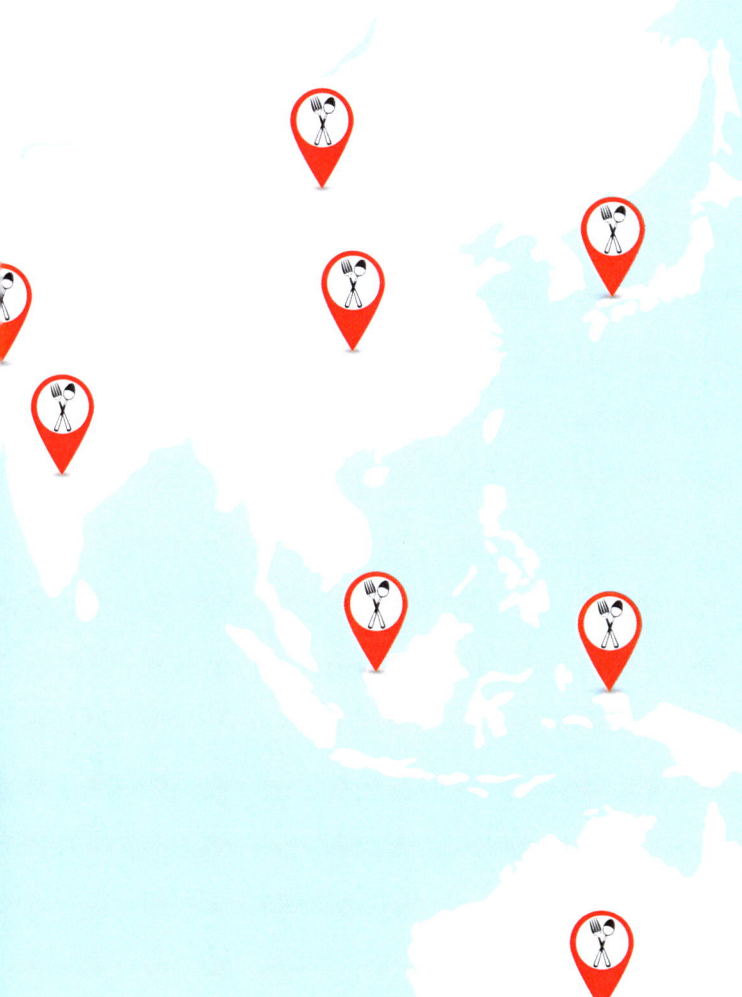

Asia &
the Pacific

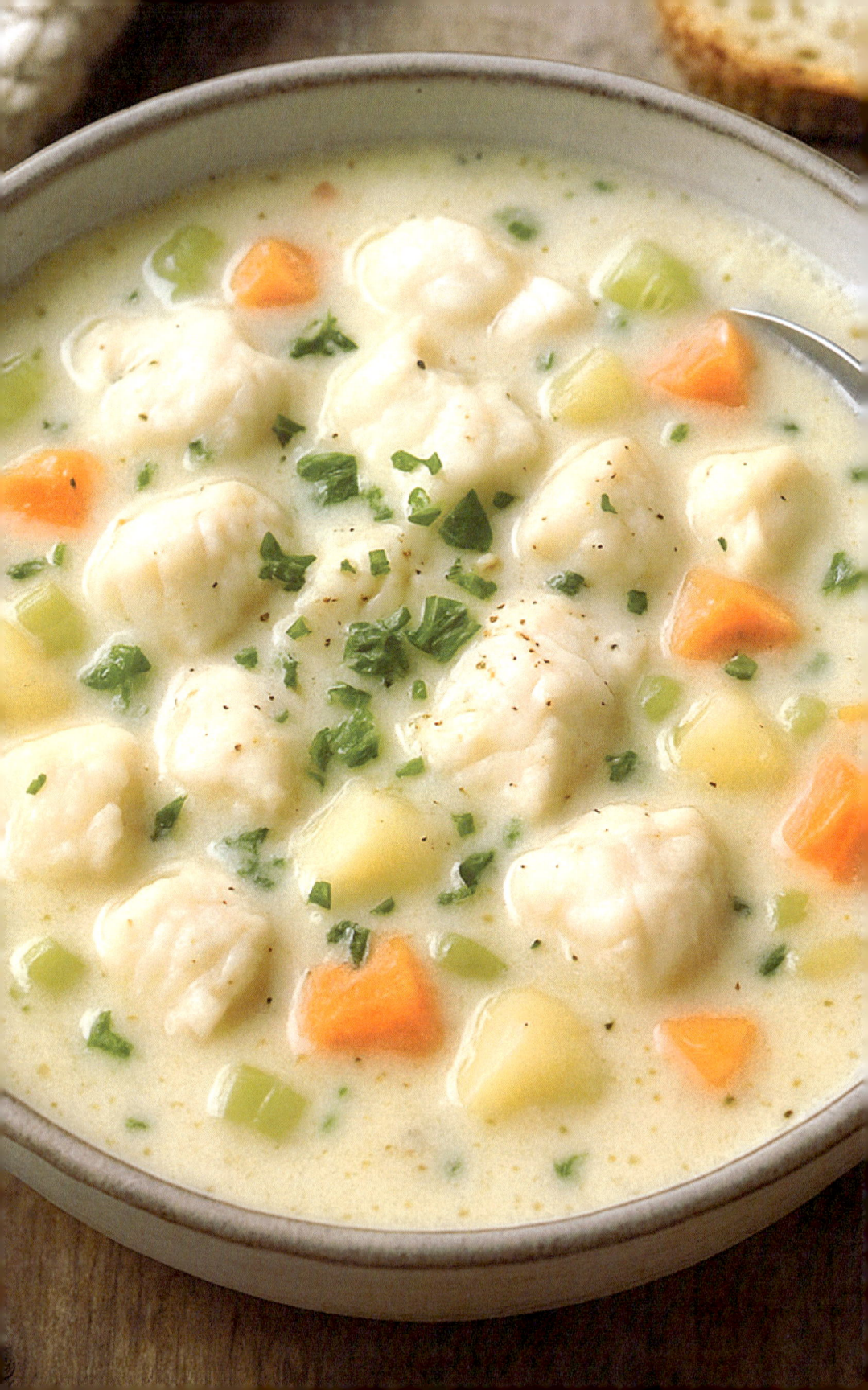

Antarctic Cozy Fish Chowder

While I love to travel in my mind, I can't say I've ever really wanted to go to Antarctica. However, if I did, I would definitely want to make a hearty fish chowder like this to keep me warm. While I doubt penguins eat this hot, creamy soup is perfect for anyone trying to keep cozy at the bottom of the world.

Ingredients:
Makes 4 servings
1 can of cooked white fish (like cod, tilapia, or halibut) — or 1 cup frozen fish, thawed
1 small onion (or 2 tablespoons dried onion flakes)
2 medium potatoes (or 1 cup frozen diced potatoes)
1 carrot (or ½ cup frozen carrots)
2 tablespoons butter or oil
2 cups milk (or 1 cup powdered milk + 2 cups water)
1 cup water or broth
Salt and pepper to taste
Optional: ½ teaspoon dried dill or thyme

Tools You'll Need:
Medium pot
Spoon
Knife (or pre-cut veggies)
Measuring cups and spoons

Tips for Accessibility:
Uses canned or frozen ingredients that store well

Warms you up from the inside out

Simple steps and minimal cleanup

Easy to scale up for teams or crews

Step-by-Step Instructions:

1 **Prepare the veggies.**
If using fresh: Peel and chop the potatoes and carrot into small chunks. Dice the onion.

2 **Cook the base.**
Put butter in the pot over medium heat. Add onion (or flakes) and stir for 2 minutes.

3 **Add veggies and liquid.**
Add potatoes, carrots, water, and a pinch of salt. Bring to a gentle boil. Cook for about 15 minutes, until veggies are soft.

4 **Add milk and fish.**
Pour in the milk and gently add the fish (break it into small pieces if needed). Add herbs if using.

5 **Simmer and season.**
Lower the heat and cook 5–10 more minutes, stirring often. Add pepper and adjust salt to taste.

6 **Serve hot.**
Spoon into bowls and enjoy! You can sprinkle a few crushed crackers on top if you like.

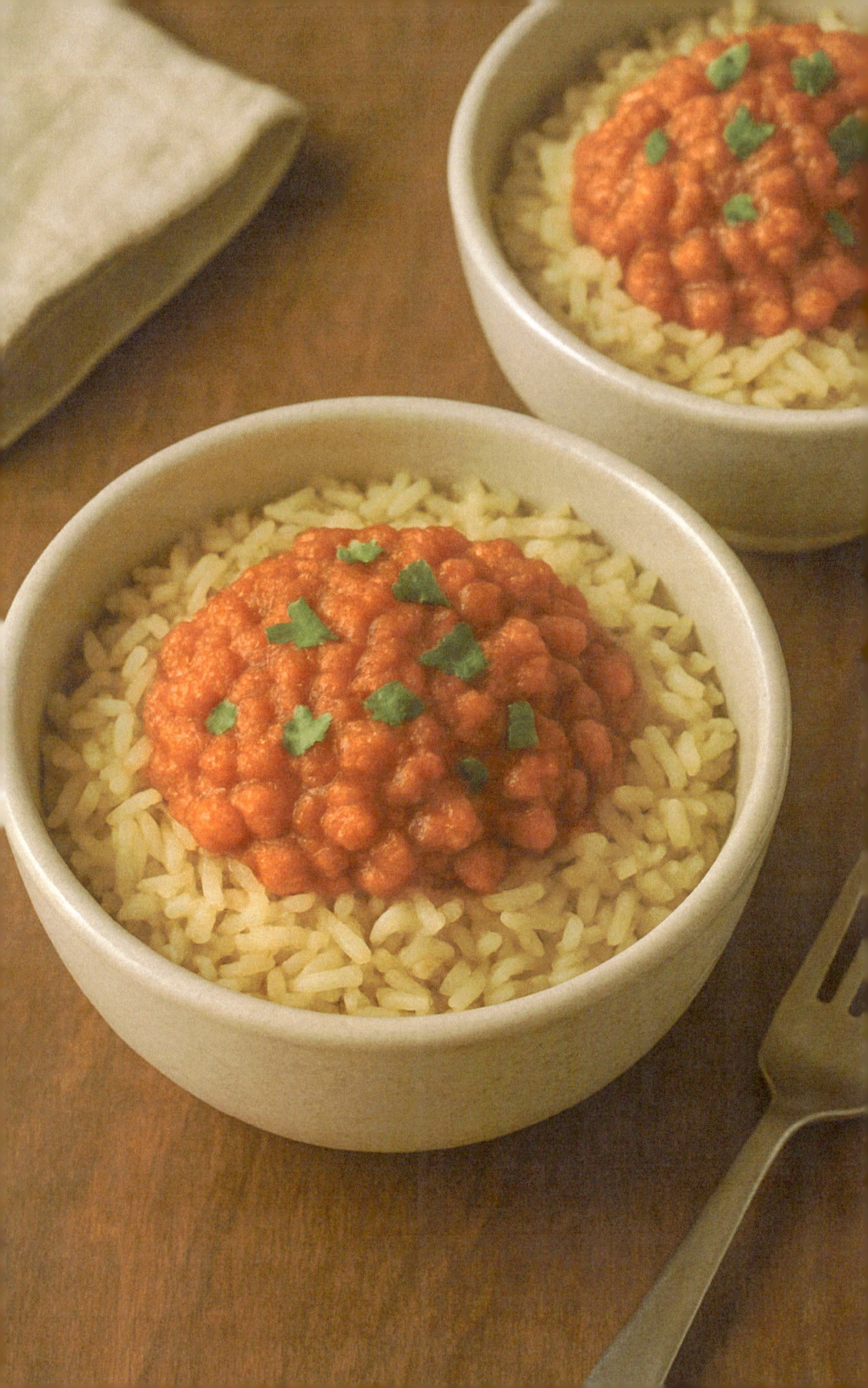

Afghan Spiced Rice & Tomato Lentil Bowls

A simple, soft dinner with fragrant spices, creamy lentils, and a tomato topping, this dish features the distinct Afghan flavors of turmeric, cumin, and mint. You can put this dish together super quickly, but the complex aroma will transport you to an authentic desert feast.

Ingredients:
Makes 2–3 servings
1 cup cooked rice (white or brown; micro-wave pouch is great)
½ cup canned lentils (rinsed and drained)
½ cup canned diced tomatoes (with juice)
1 tablespoon tomato paste or ketchup
½ teaspoon turmeric
½ teaspoon cumin (or use mild curry powder)
1 tablespoon oil or butter
A pinch of salt
Optional: 2 tablespoons plain yogurt or sour cream for topping
Optional: a sprinkle of dried mint or parsley

Tools You'll Need:
Medium pan or pot
Spoon for stirring
Bowl and spoon for serving

Tips for Accessibility:
Use canned lentils and tomatoes—no chopping required.

Microwaveable rice saves time and avoids boiling water.

Cooking involves just stirring and scooping.

The warm spices and colors offer a satisfying sensory experience.

Dish is naturally gluten-free and vegetarian.

Step-by-Step Instructions:

1 **Warm the spices.**
In a pan over medium heat, add oil or butter.
Sprinkle in turmeric and cumin. Stir gently for 30 seconds to release the aroma.

2 **Add tomatoes and lentils.**
Add diced tomatoes (with juice), tomato paste, and lentils. Stir gently.

3 **Simmer and soften.**
Let it simmer for about 5–7 minutes, stirring occasionally. The mixture should become thick and saucy. Add a pinch of salt.

4 **Add the rice.**
Stir in the cooked rice. Mix well until everything is warm and coated in sauce.

5 **Serve and enjoy.**
Spoon into bowls. Add a dollop of yogurt or a sprinkle of mint on top if desired. Eat with a spoon—everything is soft and gentle.

Aussie Beef & Sweet Potato Mash Cups

A twist on the classic Aussie meat pie—made easy in muffin tins with creamy mash on top instead of pastry. This hearty spin on the classic meat pie comes together much easier and faster than fooling with dough, but I promise you'll feel at home down under with one of these cups on your plate.

Ingredients:

Makes 6 muffin-sized portions
½ pound (about 225g) ground beef (or cooked lentils for vegetarians)
1 small onion (or 2 tbsp dried onion flakes)
1 tablespoon tomato paste or ketchup
½ teaspoon Worcestershire sauce (or a dab of Vegemite if you like!)
1 medium sweet potato, peeled and chopped (or use pre-cut frozen)
1 tablespoon butter or margarine
A pinch of salt and pepper
Optional: shredded cheese for topping

Tools You'll Need:

Frying pan
Saucepan or microwave-safe bowl (for sweet potato)
Spoon
Muffin tin or silicone cups
Fork

Step-by-Step Instructions:

1 Cook the Sweet Potato
Boil sweet potato chunks in water for about 10–12 minutes until soft. (Or microwave with a little water for 5–6 minutes.) Drain, then mash with butter and a pinch of salt.

2 Cook the Beef
In a pan, cook ground beef and onion (or flakes) over medium heat until browned. Stir in tomato paste and Worcestershire (or Vegemite). Cook for 1 more minute, then turn off the heat.

3 Fill the Cups
Grease a muffin tin or use silicone liners. Spoon beef mixture into each cup, filling about halfway. Then top with mashed sweet potato and press gently to flatten.

4 Optional Topping
Sprinkle with cheese if you like.

5 Warm It Up
Bake in the oven at 180°C (350°F) for 10–15 minutes, or microwave each one for about 1 minute to heat through and melt the cheese.

6 Cool and Serve

Let cool slightly. Use a spoon to eat, or lift out with fingers if firm enough!

Tips for Accessibility:

Pre-cut frozen sweet potatoes make it safer and faster.

Vegemite or Worcestershire gives Aussie flavor with minimal effort.

Muffin portions make serving and cleanup easy.

Everything is soft and scooped—no knives needed.

Recipe uses a few repeatable steps with hands-on satisfaction.

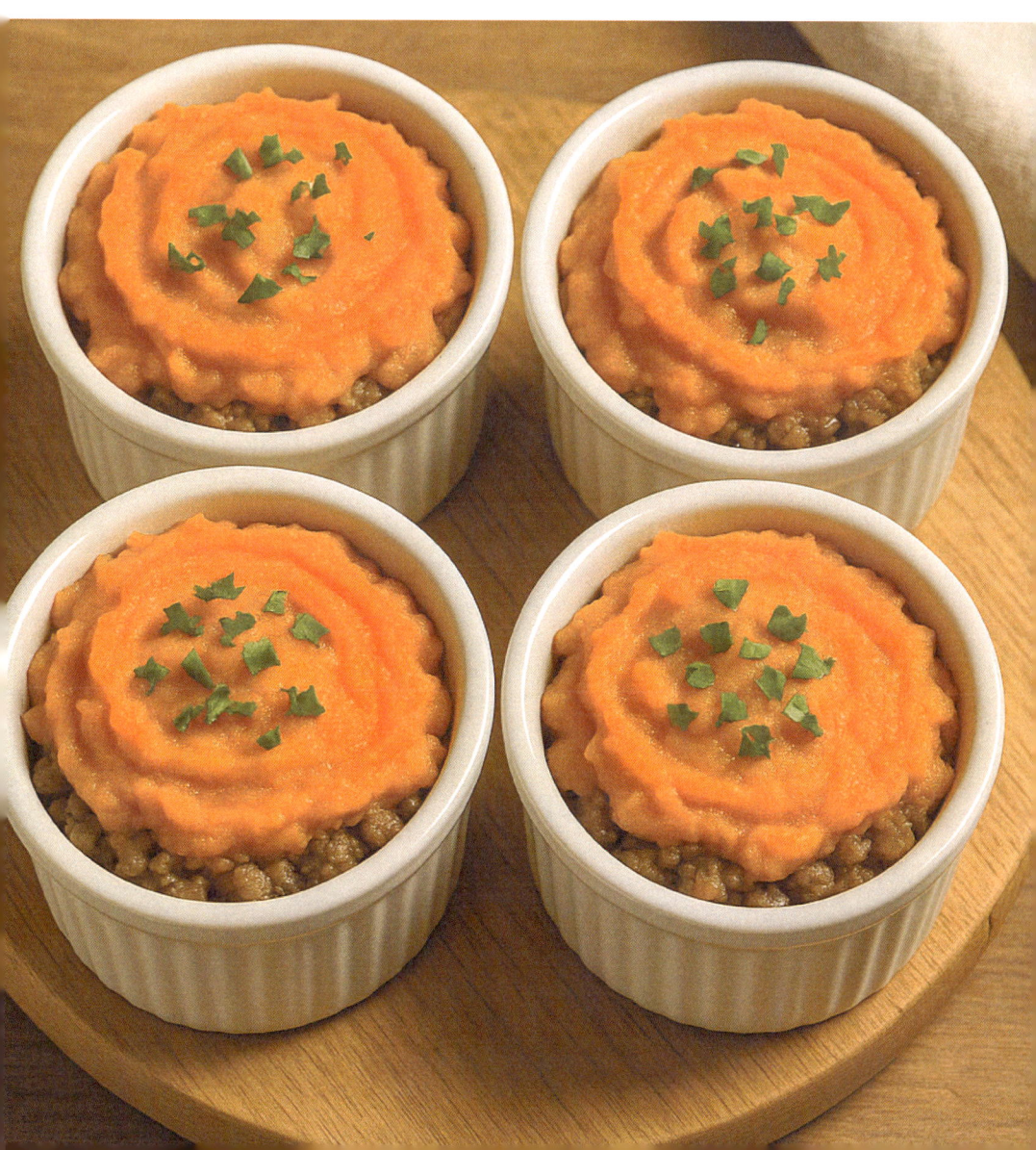

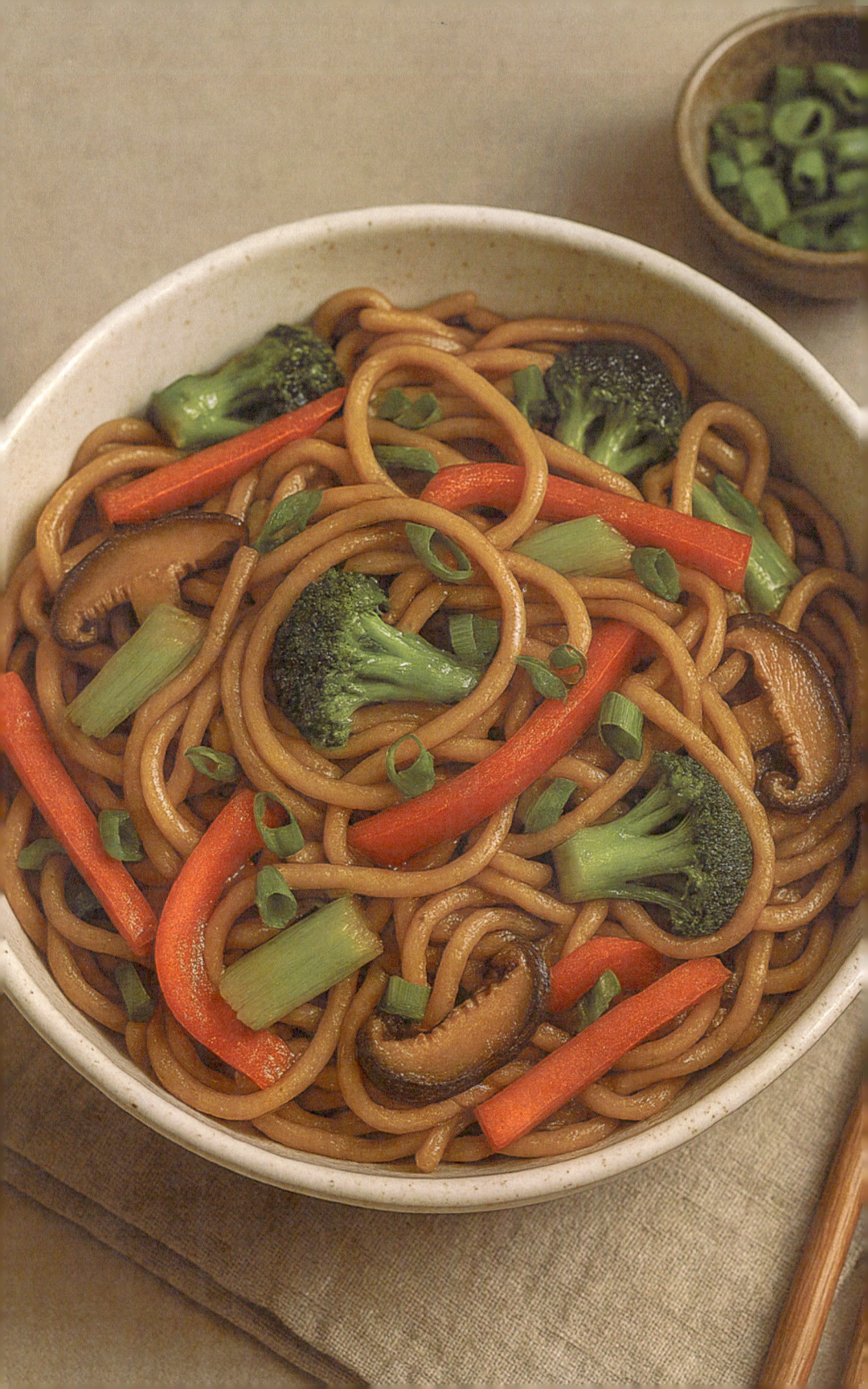

Chinese Lo Mein (Vegetarian)

This is a simple way to increase your vegetable intake. You can adjust the spices accordingly if you prefer a hotter or milder flavor. Egg noodles are what are traditionally used, but you can substitute different noodles in a pinch. You can also use whatever leftover vegetables you have on hand. This dish is typically served hot, but many people also enjoy it as a chilled leftover.

Ingredients:
8 ounces of egg noodles
1 tablespoon olive oil
2 cloves minced garlic
1 red bell pepper, sliced into thin strips
1 carrot (diced)
1 cup snow peas
2 cups broccoli

For the sauce:
2 tablespoons reduced-sodium soy sauce
(or more to taste)
2 teaspoons sugar
1 teaspoon sesame oil
½ teaspoon ground ginger
½ teaspoon Sriracha hot sauce (or more to taste)

Tools You'll Need:
Large skillet
Large pot
Measuring cups and spoons
Colander

Step-by-Step Instructions:

1 Make your sauce.
In a small bowl, mix together soy sauce, sugar, sesame oil, ginger, and Sriracha. Set aside

2 Cook your noodles.
Bring a large pot of salted water to a boil and cook noodles according to package instructions. Drain well.

3 Cook your vegetables.
Heat olive oil in a large skillet or wok over medium-high heat. Add garlic, bell paper and carrot. Cook, stirring frequently until tender, about 3 to 4 minutes. Stir in snow peas and broccoli and cook until cooked through, about 4 minutes.

4 Add noodles and sauce to skillet.
Gently toss together to combine. Serve immediately.

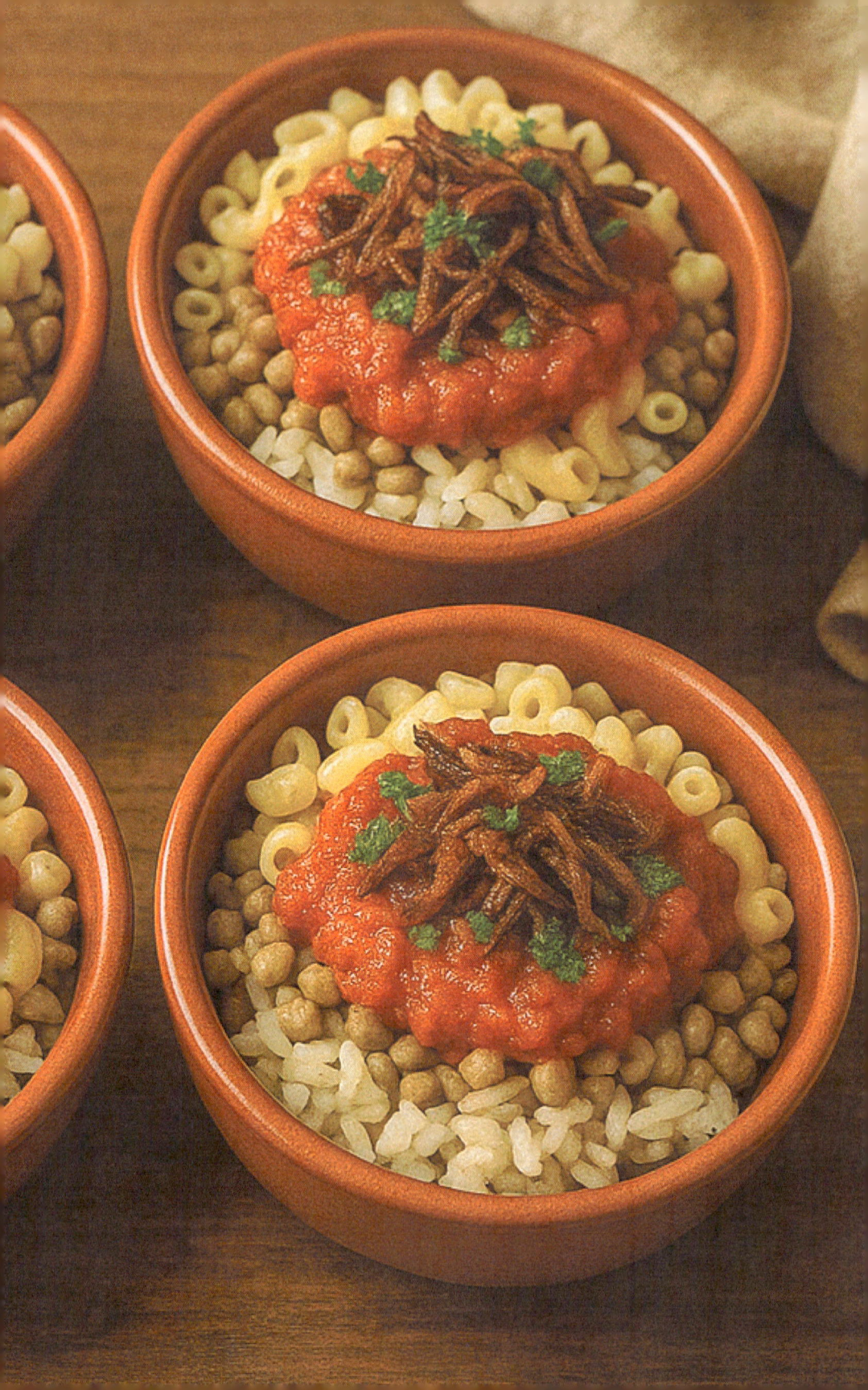

Easy Egyptian Koshari Bowls

Koshari is the national dish of Egypt and is often sold on the street. This version is streamlined by using microwavable rice, canned lentils, and optional cooked pasta, but the authentic flavors will still come through.

Ingredients:
Makes 2 servings
1 cup cooked rice (microwave pouch or leftover)
½ cup canned lentils (drained and rinsed)
½ cup canned tomato sauce or crushed tomatoes
½ teaspoon ground cumin
½ teaspoon garlic powder
1 tablespoon oil or butter
A pinch of salt
Optional: ½ cup cooked small pasta (like macaroni or mini shells)
Optional: 1 tablespoon crispy onions (store-bought)

Tools You'll Need:
Spoon
Pan or microwave-safe bowl
Serving bowl

Tips for Accessibility:
No knives or cutting required—use canned and pre-cooked ingredients.

Spoon-stirring is safe and satisfying.

Mild spices provide flavor without overwhelming the palate.

Each step uses soft ingredients that are easy to handle and chew.

Step-by-Step Instructions:

1 **Warm the base.**
In a pan (or microwave-safe bowl), combine the rice, lentils, and pasta (if using). Stir gently.

2 **Make the tomato sauce.**
Add the tomato sauce, oil or butter, cumin, garlic powder, and a pinch of salt. Stir everything together.

3 **Heat it up.**
Pan: Heat on medium for 5–6 minutes, stirring occasionally until hot.
Microwave: Heat for 2–3 minutes, stir, and heat another 1–2 minutes if needed.

4 **Serve and top.**
Scoop into bowls. Sprinkle with crispy onions if you like for added crunch and flavor.

5 **Eat and enjoy.**
Everything is soft and can be eaten easily with a spoon!

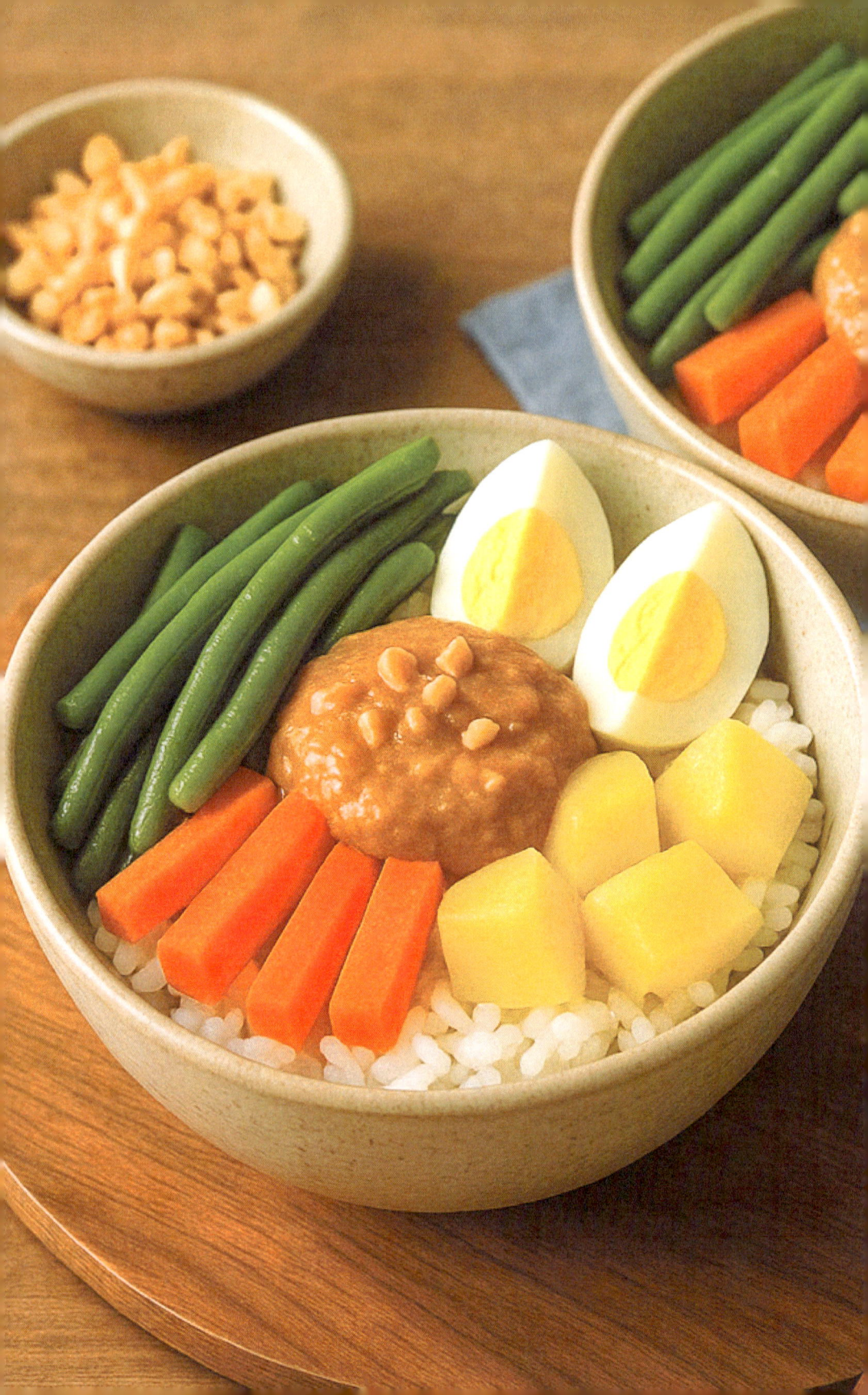

Gado-Gado Rice Bowls

Inspired by the classic Indonesian salad, Gado-Gado, these rice bowls can be made using whatever vegetables you have on hand. Almond butter can also be used in place of peanut butter if preferred. The sweet and salty sauce of Gado-Gado is what makes these bowls pop, so feel free to experiment with flavors to get just the right mix of sweet and savory to your liking.

Ingredients:
Makes 2 bowls
1 pouch (or 1 cup) cooked rice
1 cup frozen mixed vegetables (like carrots, green beans, corn, peas)
1 hard-boiled egg (store-bought or pre-made if needed)
¼ cup canned chickpeas or tofu cubes (optional protein)
2 tablespoons creamy peanut butter
1 tablespoon soy sauce
1 tablespoon warm water
1 teaspoon honey or brown sugar
Optional: 1 teaspoon lime juice

Tools You'll Need:
Microwave or pot (for veggies and rice)
Bowl and spoon
Knife (or pre-cut egg)
2 serving bowls

Tips for Accessibility:
Use pre-cooked rice and eggs for safety and speed.

Sauce is easy to mix and pour—no cooking!

Colorful veggies make it fun to assemble.

Everything can be eaten with a spoon or fork—no cutting needed at the table.

Step-by-Step Instructions:

1 Warm the Rice and Veggies
Heat the rice and frozen veggies according to package directions (usually 2–3 minutes in the microwave).
Place half the rice and veggies into each bowl.

2 Prepare the Peanut Sauce
In a small bowl, stir together peanut butter, soy sauce, warm water, and honey until smooth. Add lime juice if using. (It should be like a pourable sauce.)

3 Add the Egg and Protein
Slice the boiled egg in half (or ask for help if needed) and place on top of each bowl. Add chickpeas or tofu if using.

4 Drizzle and Serve
Spoon the peanut sauce over everything. Mix it up or leave it layered—your choice!

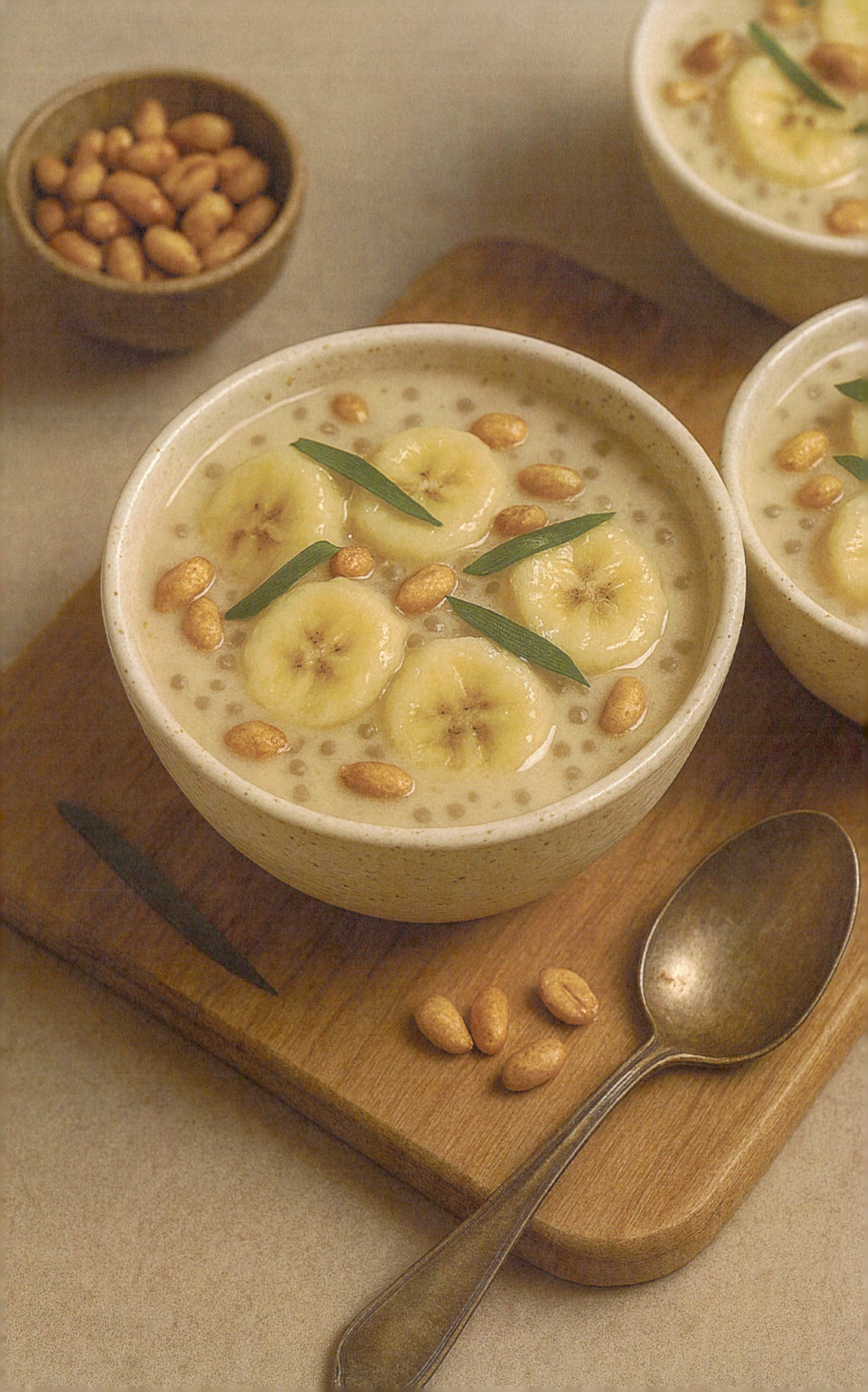

Vietnamese Chè Chuối Cups

This is a modified version of the traditional Vietnamese tapioca coconut dessert, Chè Chuối and is exceptionally sweet, creamy, and tropical. The use of tapioca pearls, which are optional in this recipe, is reminiscent of Boba tea, and they are super fun to use in your dessert making. Crushed peanuts add a bit of crunch to this dish, but you can also add shredded coconut or even some caramel syrup.

Ingredients:
Makes 4 small cups
2 ripe bananas (the softer, the better!)
1 cup canned coconut milk
2 tablespoons sugar (white or brown)
1 tablespoon small tapioca pearls (optional but fun!)
A pinch of salt
Optional: toasted sesame seeds or crushed peanuts (for topping)

Tools You'll Need:
Small saucepan
Spoon
Measuring cups and spoons
4 small cups or bowls

Tips for Accessibility:
Use pre-sliced or soft bananas to avoid cutting.

Coconut milk is poured straight from a can—no prep.

Tapioca is optional—just for texture if fun.

All steps use safe tools: no knives or ovens.

Can be eaten with a spoon and enjoyed slowly.

Step-by-Step Instructions:

1 **Cook the Tapioca (Optional)**
If using tapioca, boil it in water for 10 minutes, stirring often, until soft and clear. Drain and set aside.

2 **Make the Coconut Sauce**
In a small saucepan, add coconut milk, sugar, and a pinch of salt. Stir and heat on low for 5 minutes.

3 **Add Bananas**
Slice bananas into small circles (use a butter knife). Add them to the coconut milk. Simmer gently for 3–4 minutes, just to warm and soften the bananas.

4 **Add Tapioca (If Using)**
Stir in the tapioca pearls now. Mix gently.

5 **Serve in Cups**
Pour the warm banana-coconut mixture into small cups or bowls. Let cool for a few minutes.

6 **Top and Enjoy**
Sprinkle with sesame seeds or chopped peanuts (if using). Eat warm or chilled!

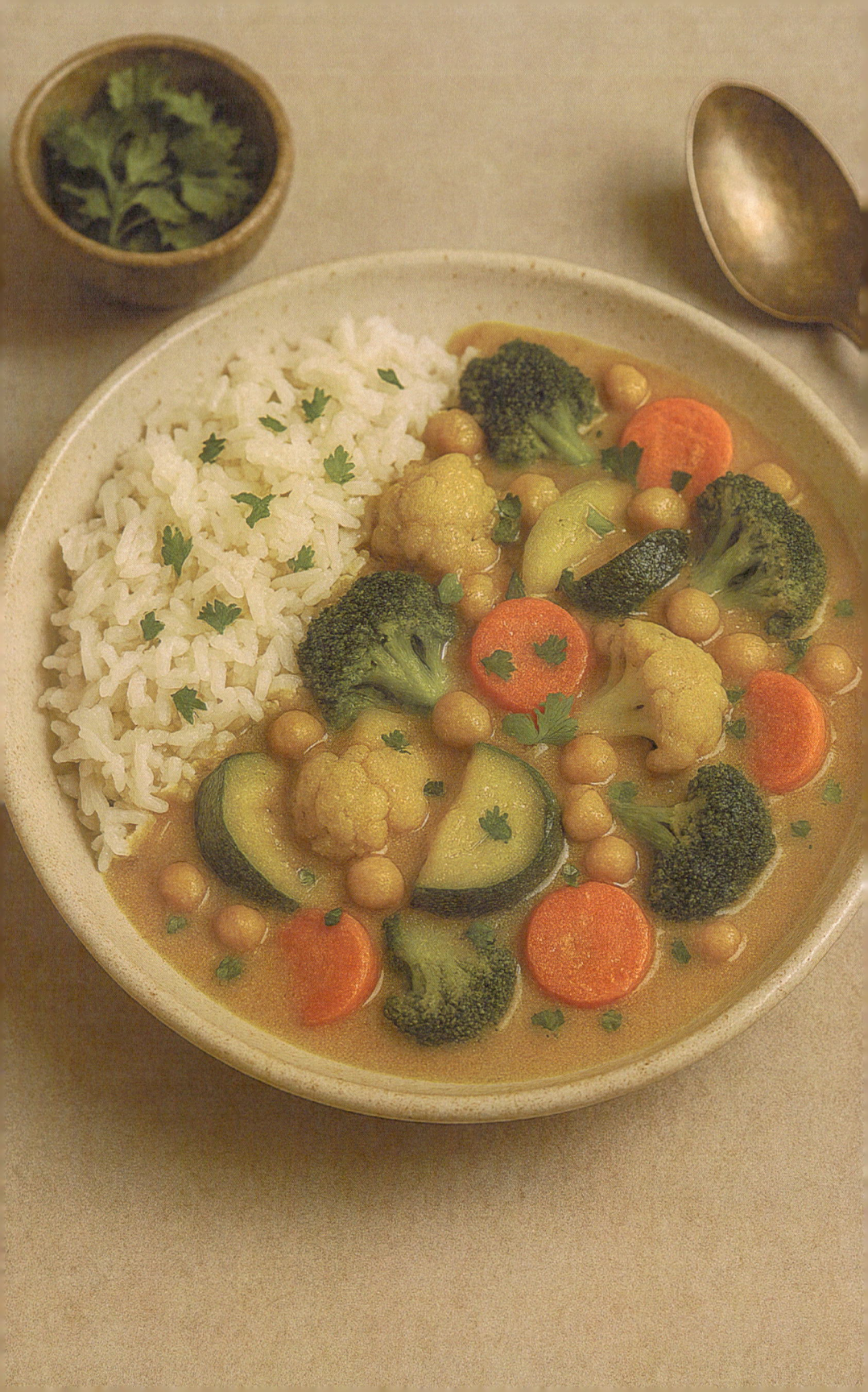

Gentle Veggie Curry with Rice

Curry dishes can be many things. Spicy, sweet, savory, mild—even creamy. This Indian veggie curry is of the creamy and mild variety. The coconut milk gives it a delicious flavor, while the traditional curry spices of turmeric and cumin up the flavor profile.

Ingredients:
Makes 2-3 servings
1 cup frozen mixed vegetables (carrots, peas, green beans, corn)
½ can (about ¾ cup) coconut milk
½ cup water
1 tablespoon tomato paste (or ketchup works too!)
½ teaspoon turmeric
½ teaspoon cumin (or curry powder)
Salt to taste
1 tablespoon oil or butter
1 pouch of microwaveable rice (or 1 cup pre-cooked rice)

Tools You'll Need:
Medium pan or pot
Spoon for stirring
Measuring spoon
Bowl or plate for serving

Tips for Accessibility:
No chopping: frozen veggies are ready to use.
All cooking is done in one pan.
Microwave rice avoids boiling water.

Step-by-Step Instructions:

1 **Cook the veggies.**
Add oil to a pan on medium heat. Pour in frozen vegetables and stir for 3–4 minutes until they start to soften.

2 **Add flavor.**
Add turmeric, cumin (or curry powder), and tomato paste. Stir for 30 seconds to mix.

3 **Make it saucy.**
Pour in the coconut milk and water. Stir everything gently. Bring to a light simmer (small bubbles). Let it cook for 5–8 minutes until the veggies are soft and the sauce is creamy.

4 **Warm the rice.**
Heat the rice in the microwave according to package instructions or use leftover cooked rice.

5 **Serve and enjoy.**
Spoon some rice into a bowl or plate. Pour the veggie curry on top of or next to it. Eat with a spoon or fork.

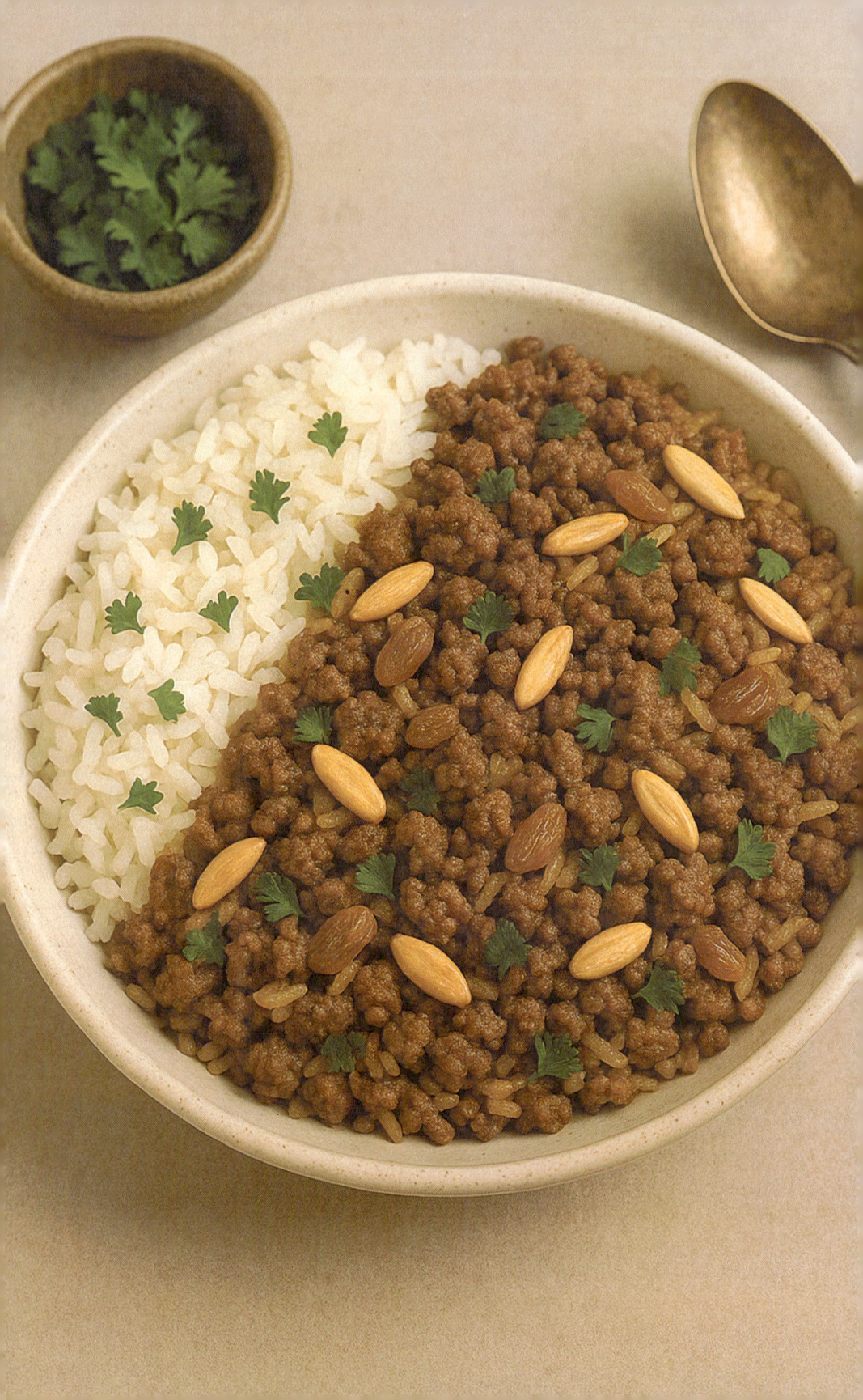

Iraqi Spiced Rice & Beef Bowls

A soft and comforting dinner with seasoned beef, warm rice, and a hint of cinnamon, these bowls are super easy to put together. It's well worth it to top with hummus for an authentic Iraqi beef bowl, and the addition of raisins or dates helps temper the salty with the sweet.

Ingredients:
Makes 2-3 servings

1 cup cooked rice (microwave pouch or pre-cooked)

½ pound ground beef (or ground chicken or lentils)

½ teaspoon ground cinnamon

½ teaspoon turmeric

½ teaspoon cumin

1 tablespoon oil or butter

Salt to taste

Optional: 2 tablespoons plain yogurt or hummus for topping

Optional: a spoonful of raisins or chopped dates for sweetness

Tools You'll Need:
Pan

Spoon for stirring

Bowl and spoon for serving

Tips for Accessibility:
Ground beef requires no chopping and cooks quickly.

Microwave rice avoids boiling water and simplifies timing.

All steps involve stirring and scooping—no sharp tools.

Cinnamon and turmeric add aroma, color, and warmth without heat.

Yogurt and raisins offer soft, sensory-friendly toppings.

Step-by-Step Instructions:

1 **Cook the beef.**
Put oil in a pan over medium heat. Add ground beef. Stir with a spoon and cook for 5–7 minutes until browned and fully cooked.

2 **Add spices.**
Sprinkle in cinnamon, turmeric, cumin, and a pinch of salt. Stir for 1 minute so the spices coat the meat.

3 **Mix in the rice.**
Add the cooked rice to the pan. Stir until everything is mixed and warm (about 2 more minutes). Turn off the heat.

4 **Serve and top.**
Spoon the rice and beef into a bowl. Add a dollop of yogurt or hummus on top. Sprinkle raisins or chopped dates if you want a touch of sweetness.

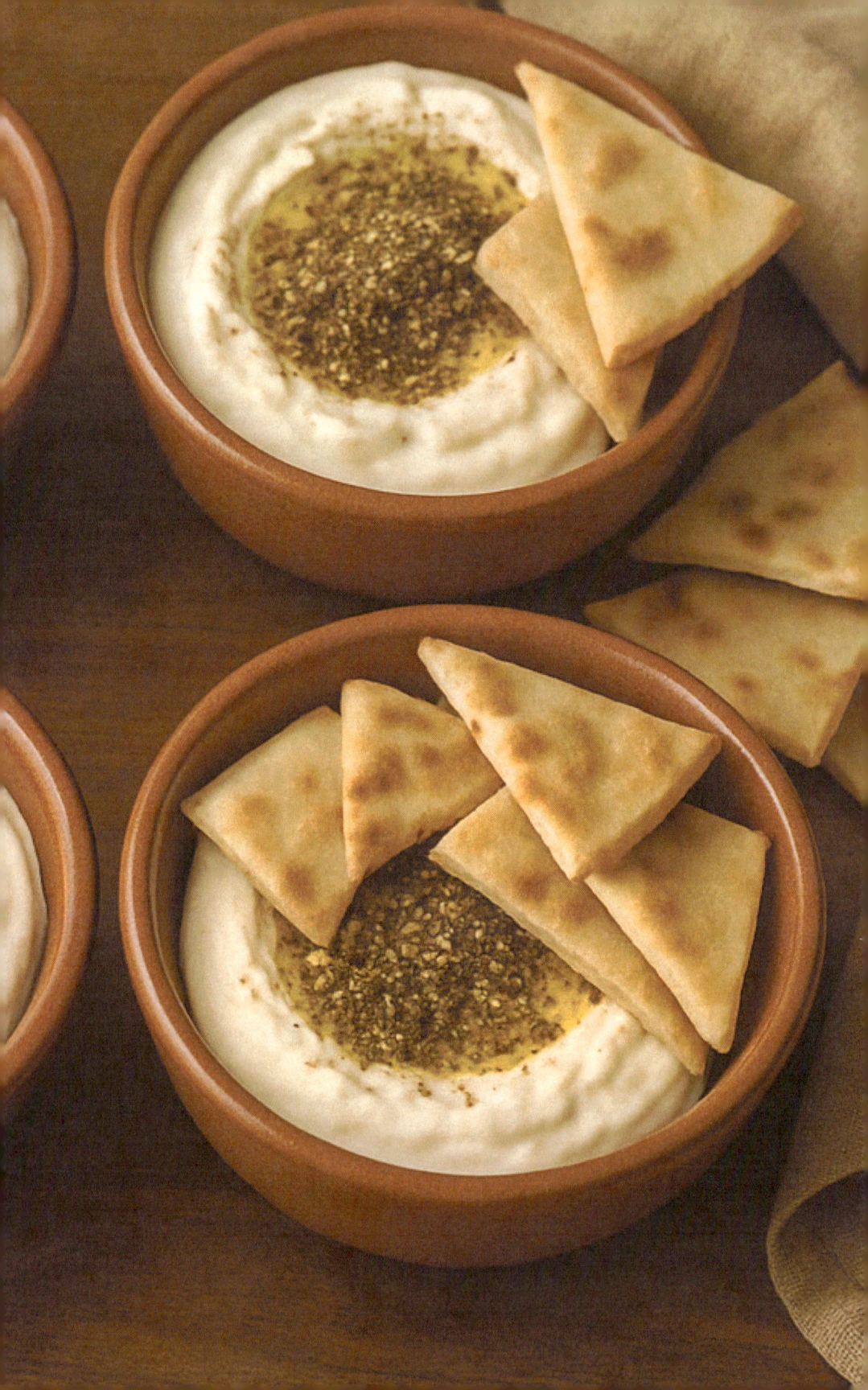

Lebanese Labneh & Za'atar Pita Scoops

In Lebanese culture, forks are often replaces with pita for scooping up delicious bits of sauces and creamy spreads like hummus or Lebanese Labneh, which is a soft cheese similar to yogurt. This is a great meal for when it's too hot to cook or you want something filling fast.

Ingredients:
½ cup labneh (or plain Greek yogurt, strained)
1 tablespoon olive oil
1 teaspoon za'atar spice blend
1 tablespoon chopped black olives (or tapenade – optional)
1 soft pita bread (or 2 mini pitas)
Optional: 1 tablespoon cucumber (pre-chopped) for extra crunch

Tools You'll Need:
Spoon
Small bowl
Toaster oven or pan
Plate

Step-by-Step Instructions:

1 **Make the dip.**
In a small bowl, stir together the labneh, olive oil, and za'atar. Add chopped olives or cucumber if using. Mix until smooth and creamy.

2 **Warm the pita.**
Toast the pita in a toaster oven or warm it in a dry pan for about 1 minute per side—just until soft and bendable. (You can skip this if the pita is already soft and fresh.)

3 **Cut or tear the pita.**
Tear the warm pita into triangle shapes or strips. Use clean hands or ask for help cutting if needed.

4 **Scoop and serve.**
Place the labneh dip in the center of a plate and surround it with the pita pieces. Use the pita to scoop the dip—no spoon or fork needed!

Tips for Accessibility:
Labneh is soft and easy to mix—no stove or knife required.

Tearing pita by hand makes it a fun and safe sensory activity.

All ingredients are soft, spoonable, and visually appealing.

Can be eaten entirely with fingers—no utensils required for serving or eating.

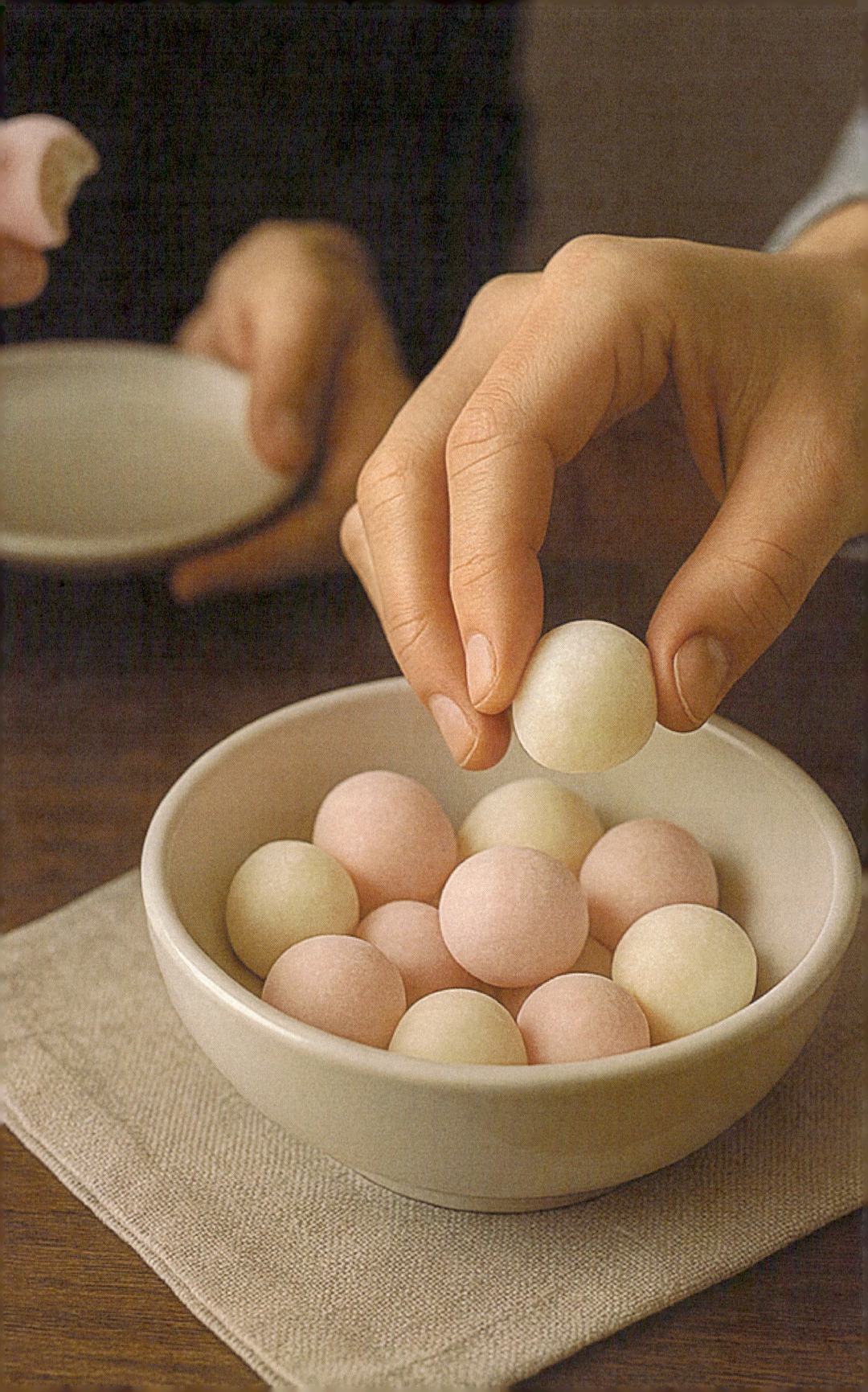

Mochi Yogurt Bites

Mochi is a traditional Japanese frozen dessert using glutinous rice (mochiko) that is soaked and then pounded into balls and filled with paste or ice cream. These bites use yogurt instead of ice cream, but once chilled you won't be able to tell the difference. They are sweet little explosions in your mouth.

Ingredients:
Makes about 10–12 bites
1 cup plain or flavored yogurt (strawberry, vanilla, or matcha are great!)
2 tablespoons honey or maple syrup
½ cup glutinous rice flour (also called mochiko – found in Asian stores)
⅓ cup water
Cornstarch or potato starch (for dusting)
Optional: small pieces of fruit (like banana, strawberry, or canned mandarin)

Tools You'll Need:
Microwave-safe bowl
Spoon
Small tray or plate
Plastic wrap
Sifter or clean shaker for cornstarch

Tips for Accessibility:
All mixing is done with a spoon—no sharp tools.

Microwave replaces stovetop for safety.

Dusting with cornstarch makes it easy to handle.

Use a mini ice cream scoop or wet spoon for easier shaping.

Great for sensory exploration: soft, squishy, sweet, and cold!

Step-by-Step Instructions:

1 **Make the mochi mixture.**
In a microwave-safe bowl, mix the rice flour, yogurt, water, and honey. Stir until smooth—like a pancake batter.

2 **Cook the mochi base.**
Cover loosely with plastic wrap. Microwave for 1 minute. Stir with a spoon. Microwave again for 30–60 seconds, until it becomes thick and sticky like dough.

3 **Cool and shape.**
Let the mochi cool a bit. Dust a plate or tray with cornstarch. Scoop small spoonfuls of the warm mochi onto the tray. If it's too sticky, dust your hands with more starch and gently shape into round bites.

4 **Add fruit (optional).**
You can press a small piece of soft fruit into the center of each ball if you like.

5 **Chill and enjoy**
Put in the fridge for 30 minutes. Then eat with your fingers or a spoon!

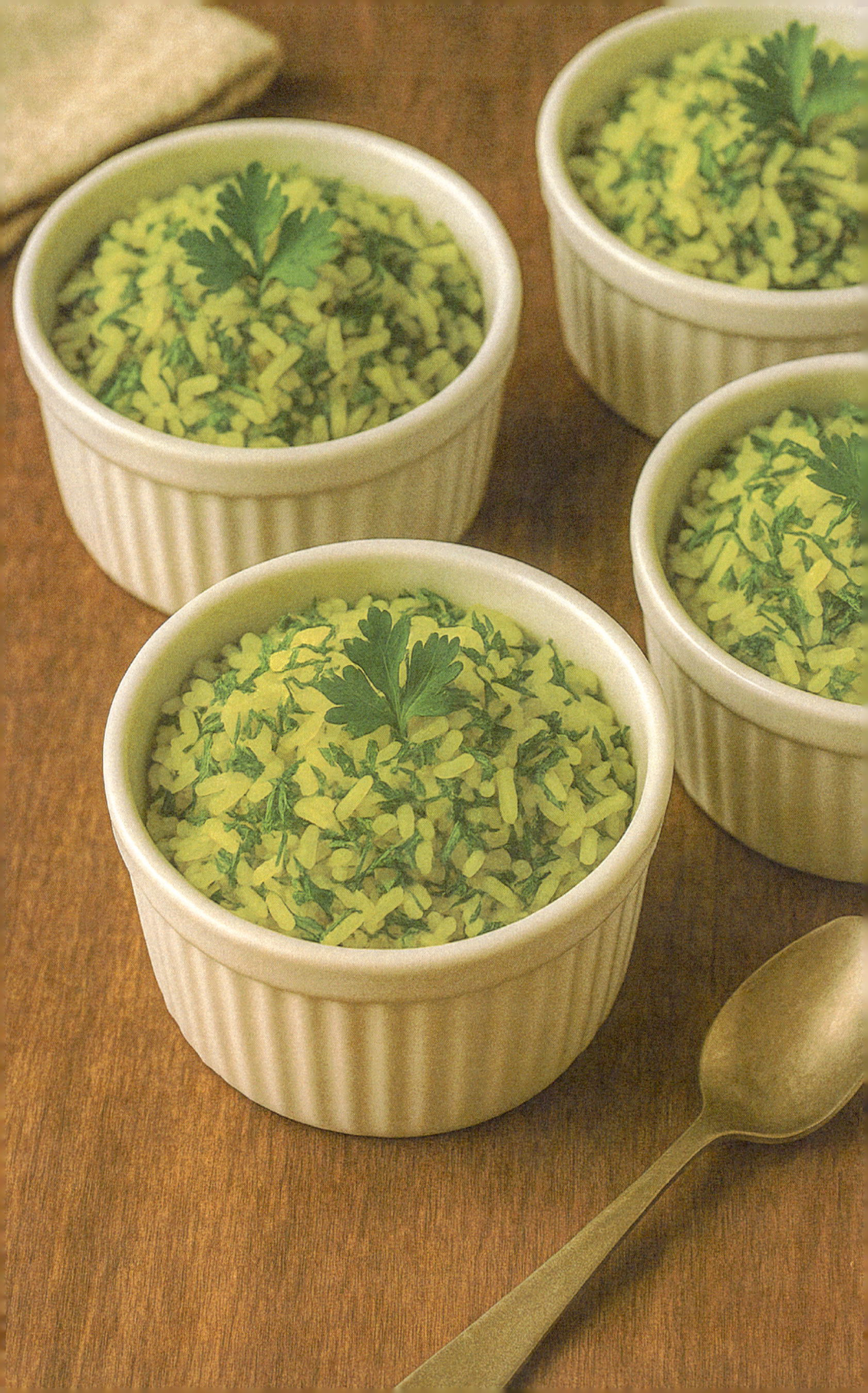

Persian Golden Rice & Herb Cups

Tahdig means "bottom of the pot" in Farsi, and refers to that crispy bit of rice that often sticks to the bottom of a pan after it is cooked. These cups will get that same crunchy deliciousness by oiling the muffin tins before putting them in the oven. The turmeric gives these herby cups a distinct golden hue, just like what I imagine a Persian sunset must be like.

Ingredients:
Makes 6 muffin-size cups – 2 servings
1 ½ cups cooked white rice (from pouch or pre-cooked)
2 tablespoons plain yogurt
1 egg
1 tablespoon chopped fresh or dried herbs (dill, parsley, or mint)
½ teaspoon turmeric (for golden color)
A pinch of salt
1 tablespoon oil or butter (for brushing)
Optional: a few raisins or barberries for sweetness

Tools You'll Need:
Mixing bowl
Spoon
Muffin tin or silicone baking cups
Oven or toaster oven

Tips for Accessibility:
Use microwave rice for ease.

Pre-chopped herbs or dried herbs make it simpler.

Muffin cups help with portioning and eliminate slicing.

All mixing is done with a spoon—no sharp tools needed.

Visual and tactile satisfaction—golden color, soft center, crisp edge.

Step-by-Step Instructions:

1 Preheat oven.
   Set oven or toaster oven to 180°C (350°F).

2 Mix everything together.
   In a bowl, stir rice, yogurt, egg, herbs, turmeric, and salt. Mix well until it's bright yellow and slightly sticky.

3 Grease the pan
   Brush muffin tin or cups with oil or butter so the bottoms get crispy.

4 Fill and press.
   Spoon the rice mixture into each muffin cup. Press down gently with the back of a spoon to pack it in.

5 Bake the cups.
   Bake for 20–25 minutes until the bottoms are golden and edges are slightly crispy.

6 Cool and serve.
   Let them cool for 5 minutes. Use a spoon to lift each rice cup onto a plate. Sprinkle with raisins or serve with a dollop of yogurt on the side.

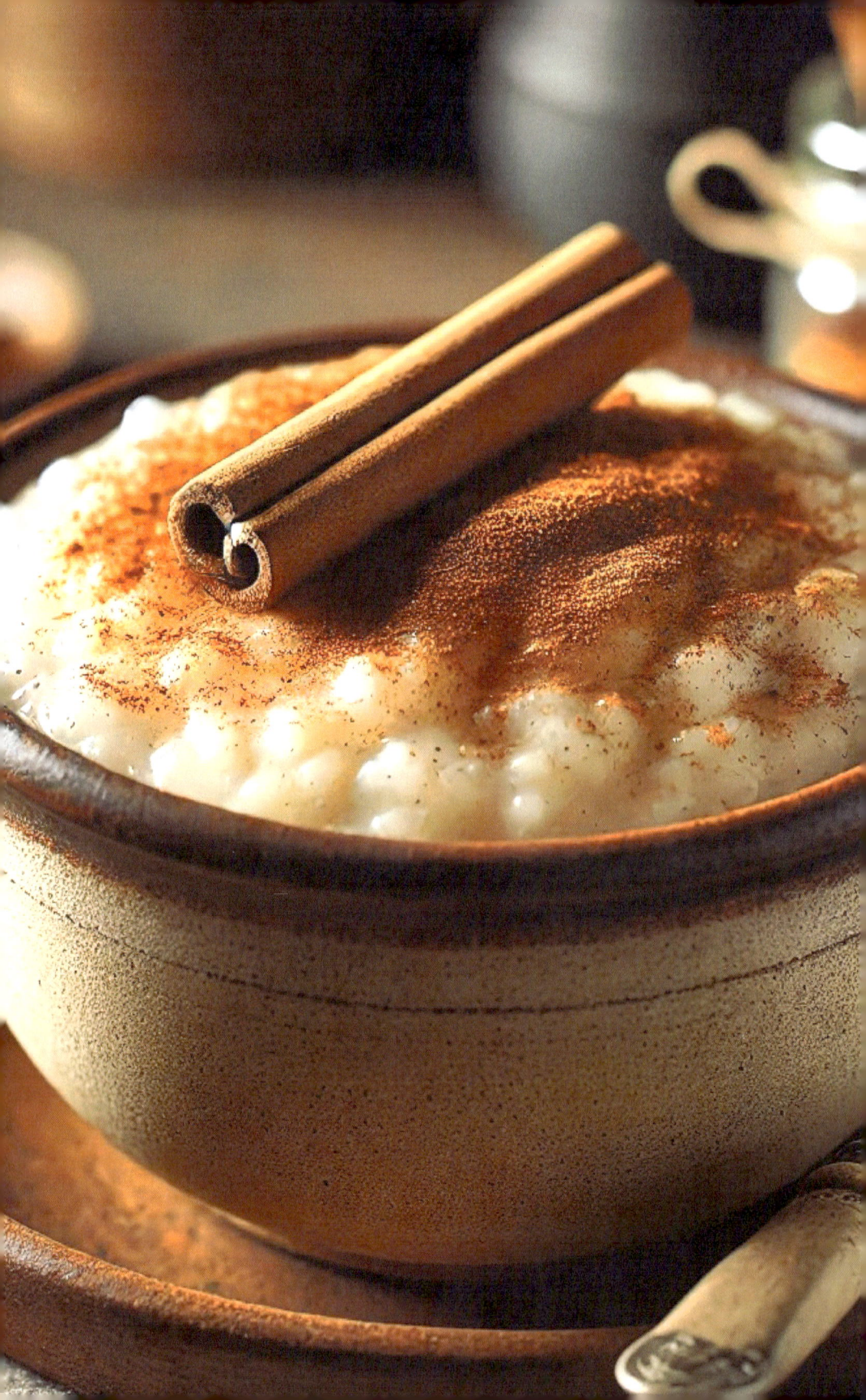

Rice Pudding

Rice pudding is great as both a dessert and for breakfast. Add raisins, chocolate chips, or shredded coconut on top for visual flair and extra sweetness. If you prefer a dairy-free option, opt for a higher-fat milk alternative, such as coconut or soy milk, for the best flavor. Don't leave your rice pudding as it is cooking, and make sure to stir often so it doesn't burn!

Ingredients:
1 ½ cup white rice
1 cinnamon stick
½ gallon of milk (whole or low fat, but non-dairy options work too)
½ cup sugar (or slightly more if you like yours extra sweet)
Optional: ½ cup shredded coconut, raisins, or chocolate chips for topping

Tools You'll Need:
Medium pot
Measuring cups and spoons
Spatula or wooden spoon

Step-by-Step Instructions:

1 Bring your rice to a boil.
   In a medium pot add your water and cinnamon stick and bring to a boil. Add your rice and when it starts boiling again add your milk and sugar.

2 Make your pudding.
   Keep your water to a slow, rolling boil and stir often as your rice cooks and the pudding begins to form. Make sure to keep the sides from sticking, or it will burn. Continue to stir for roughly 30 to 45 minutes or until the proper consistency is reached, then remove from the heat and let sit for 5 minutes before serving. Spoon into bowls and sprinkle on toppings if desired.

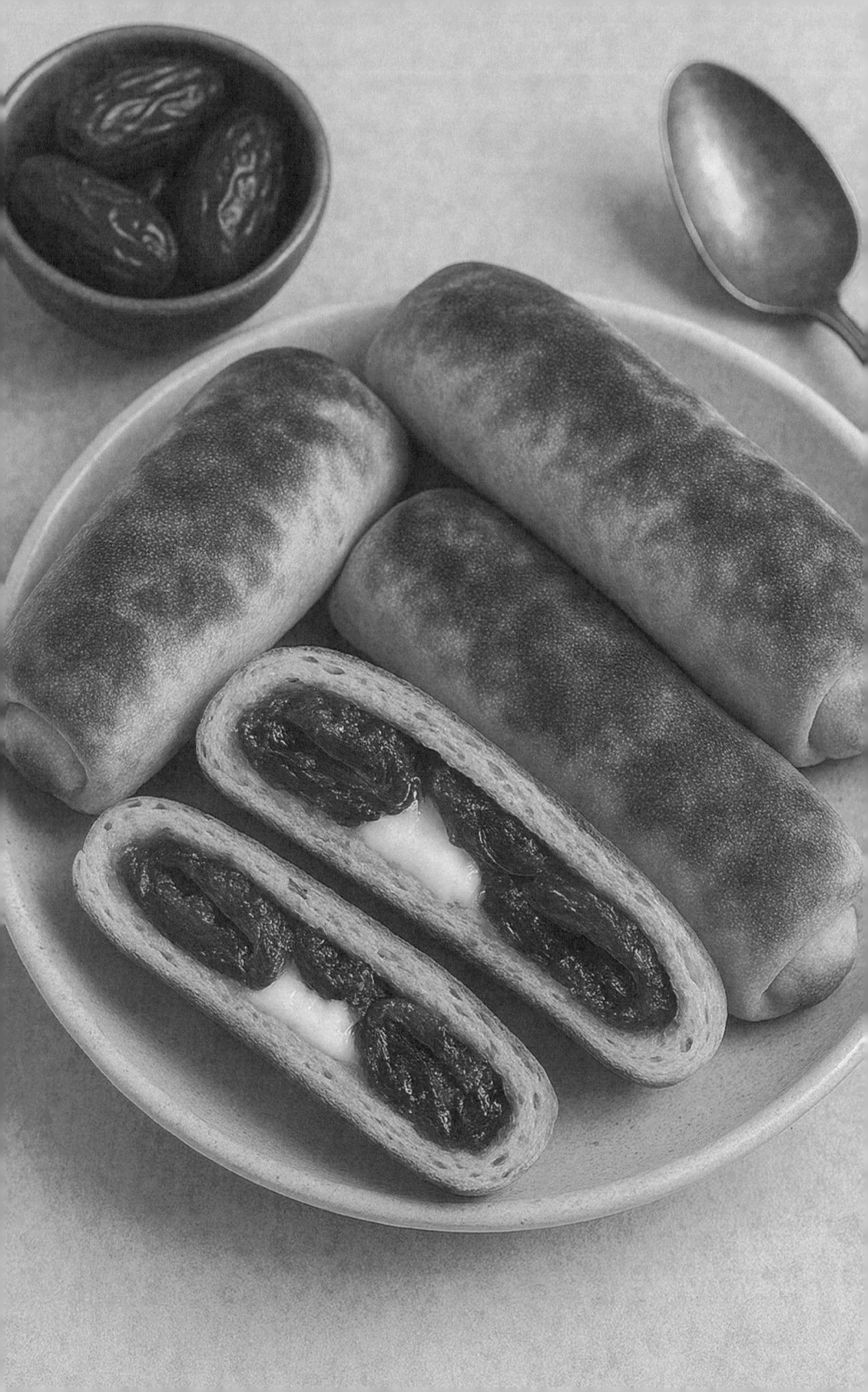

Saudi Date & Cheese Flatbread Rolls

Dates are an important part of Middle Eastern cuisine. These sweet, versatile chewy bites are high in antioxidants and fiber, and are particularly delicious when filled with a soft cheese, wrapped in bacon and put in the oven. These flatbread rolls are like little date and cheese pizzas. The pistachios and honey add a great authentic kick to this all-around knockout appetizer.

Ingredients:
Makes 6 mini rolls
2 soft flour or whole wheat tortillas (or flatbread)
6 pitted dates (Medjool or any soft kind)
3 tablespoons cream cheese or soft white cheese
½ teaspoon cinnamon
1 tablespoon plain yogurt or honey (optional topping)
Optional: A pinch of sesame seeds or crushed pistachios

Tools You'll Need:
Spoon
Fork (optional for mashing dates)
Small bowl
Plate

Tips for Accessibility:
All ingredients are soft and safe—no sharp tools or heat required.

Mixing, spreading, and rolling are tactile, enjoyable tasks.

Dates can be mashed by hand for fun sensory feedback.

Wraps are easy to hold and eat with fingers—no cutting needed at the table.

Step-by-Step Instructions:

1 **Mash the dates.**
 Place the pitted dates in a small bowl. Use a fork or clean fingers to mash them until soft and spreadable. Add a pinch of cinnamon and stir.

2 **Spread the cheese.**
 Lay the tortillas flat. Use a spoon to spread cream cheese evenly over the surface.

3 **Add the date mix.**
 Spread the mashed dates on top of the cheese. Use the back of the spoon to gently smooth it out.

4 **Roll and slice.**
 Carefully roll the tortillas up like a log. Then use your hands to press them gently into place. Cut into 3 mini rolls each using a butter knife or ask for help if needed.

5 **Top and serve.**
 Place rolls on a plate. Drizzle with a little yogurt or honey, and sprinkle with sesame seeds or pistachios if using. Eat with fingers or a fork!

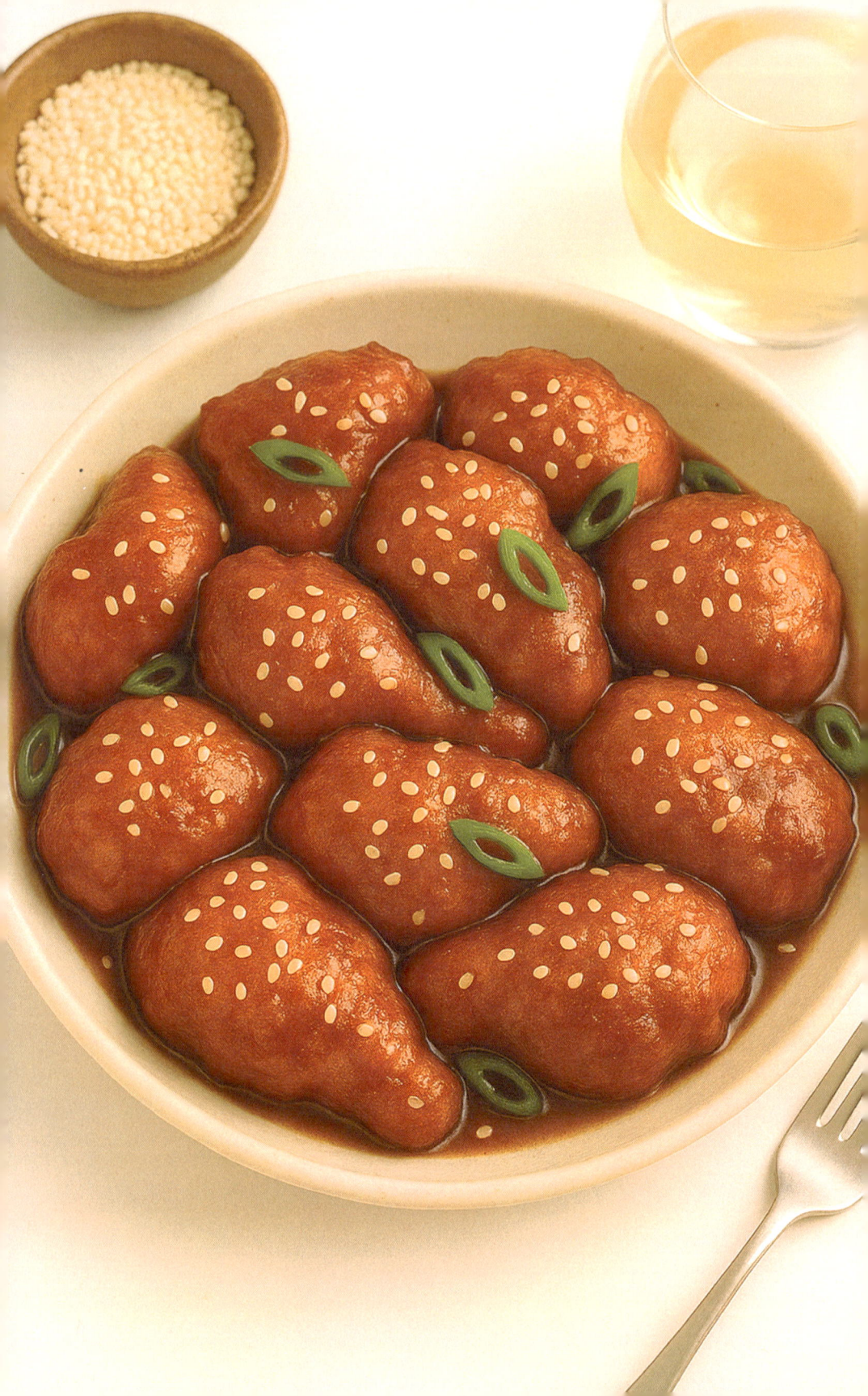

Sticky Korean Chicken

Korean chicken is a hit for a reason. The perfect mix of sweet honey and salty soy sauce (plus a dash of heat) make this dish absolutely delicious—and a little messy to eat! Serve them with rice or noodles for a full meal.

Ingredients:

3 pounds of chicken legs or thighs (bone in, skin on)
4 green onions (sliced)
½ cup honey
1 tablespoon vegetable oil
¼ cup soy sauce
4 cloves of garlic (minced)
1 tablespoon grated ginger
1 teaspoon red chili flakes
Optional: ¼ cup sesame seeds

Tools You'll Need:

Large bowl
Shallow dish
Measuring cups and spoons
Plastic wrap
Tongs
Basting brush
Meat thermometer
Parchment paper

Step-by-Step Instructions:

1 **Make the sauce and marinate the chicken.**
In a large bowl, mix honey, soy sauce, ginger, garlic, oil, and red chili flakes. Place chicken in a shallow dish and pour over the sauce. Turn chicken over in the sauce a few times to make sure it's coated, then cover dish with plastic wrap or a lid and marinate it in the refrigerator for at least two hours.

2 **Preheat oven to 375 degrees F and line a baking pan or dish with parchment paper.**
Remove the chicken from the refrigerator and use tongs to remove the chicken and place it in the parchment-lined baking dish. Keep the marinade.

3 **Bake your chicken.**
Cook the chicken in the oven for 20 minutes, then remove and brush with marinade and return to the oven, baking until juices run clear and the internal temperature reaches 180 degrees F.

4 **Remove from oven.**
Sprinkle sliced green onions and sesame seeds, if using, and serve alongside rice or noodles.

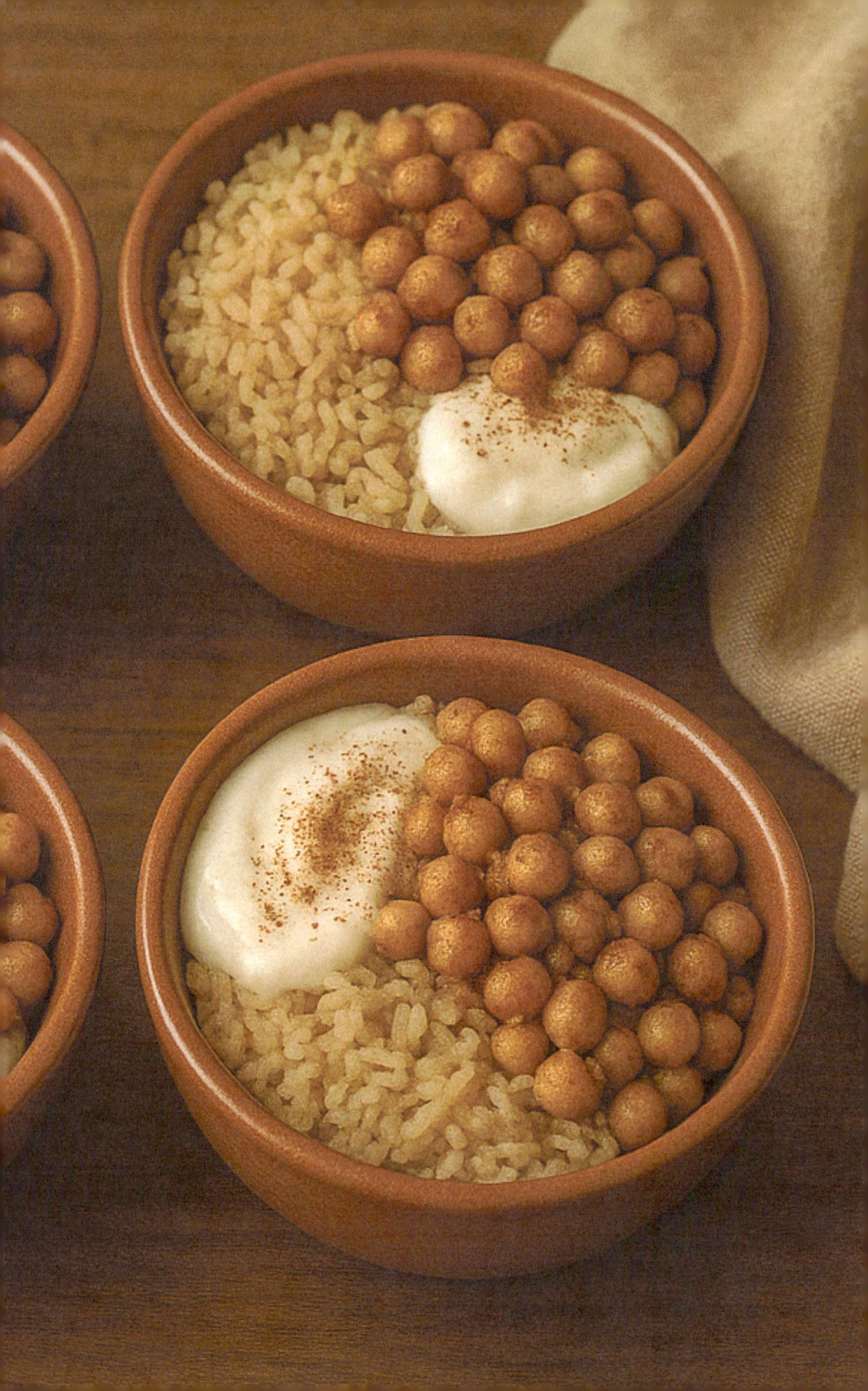

Syrian Cinnamon Rice Bowls with Chickpeas & Yogurt

A cozy, scoopable dinner with spiced rice, tender chickpeas, and a creamy yogurt drizzle—no frying, no sharp tools, and full of Middle Eastern flavor. Syrian cuisine is a great blend of Middle Eastern and Mediterranean influences, which you'll see here with the mix of chickpeas and yogurt with cinnamon and mint.

Ingredients:
Makes 2–3 servings
1 cup cooked white rice (microwave pouch or pre-cooked)
½ cup canned chickpeas (drained and rinsed)
½ teaspoon ground cinnamon
1 tablespoon olive oil or butter
Salt to taste
½ cup plain yogurt (for topping)
Optional: 1 tablespoon chopped parsley or mint (fresh or dried)
Optional: 1 tablespoon raisins or pine nuts

Tools You'll Need:
Medium pan or microwave-safe bowl
Spoon
Serving bowl or plate

Tips for Accessibility:
Microwave rice and canned chickpeas reduce cooking steps.

Cinnamon and yogurt add gentle flavor without heat.

All steps involve scooping and stirring—no cutting or measuring with precision.

Soft and nourishing textures are easy to chew and digest.

Toppings allow creativity and visual satisfaction.

Step-by-Step Instructions:

1 **Heat the rice and chickpeas.**
In a pan, add a spoon of olive oil or butter. Add the rice and chickpeas. Stir gently and warm for about 5 minutes on medium heat (or microwave in a bowl for 2–3 minutes).

2 **Add flavor.**
Sprinkle in cinnamon and a pinch of salt. Stir until everything is combined and aromatic. Turn off the heat.

3 **Serve in bowls.**
Scoop the warm rice and chickpea mix into bowls. Add a spoonful of yogurt on top.

4 **Top it off (Optional).**
Sprinkle with parsley, raisins, or pine nuts for extra flavor and color.

5 **Eat and enjoy.**
Everything can be eaten with a spoon. Serve warm or room temperature.

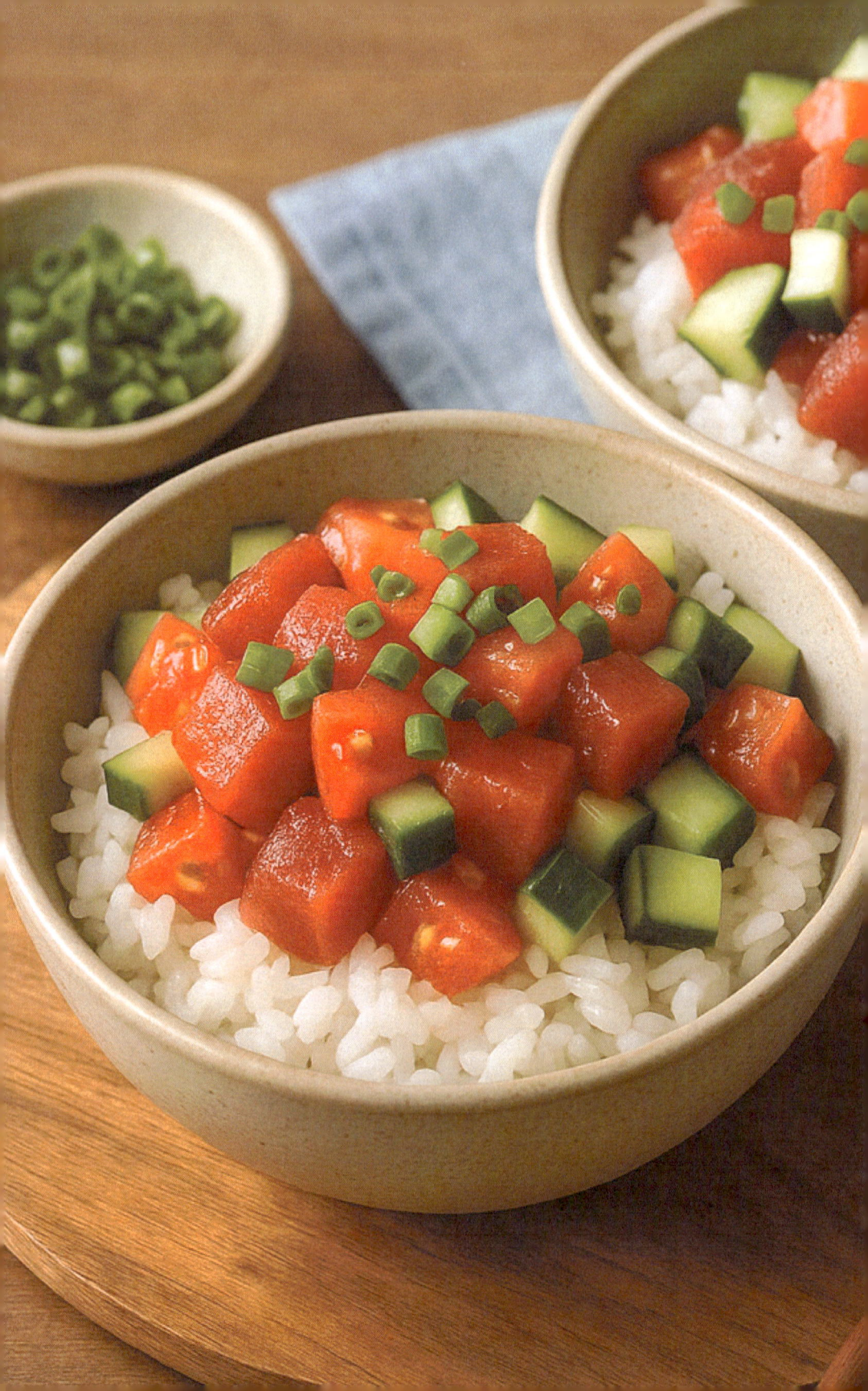

Tahitian Tuna Rice Bowls (Inspired by Poisson Cru)

This simplified, tropical-style rice bowl with tuna, coconut, and fruit is a spin on the national dish of French Polynesia, Poisson Cru, which is similar to ceviche. The tropical sweetness of the coconut and pineapple pair well with the tuna. Close your eyes and imagine you're on a white sand beach somewhere snacking on this.

Ingredients:
Makes 2 bowls
1 pouch (or 1 cup) of cooked white or brown rice
1 small can of tuna (in water or oil, drained)
¼ cup canned pineapple (chopped small) or mango pieces
¼ cup shredded carrot (fresh or pre-shredded)
2 tablespoons canned coconut milk
1 teaspoon lime juice (optional)
A pinch of salt
Optional: a sprinkle of green onion or chopped cucumber

Tools You'll Need:
Mixing bowl
Spoon
Can opener (if needed)
2 serving bowls

Step-by-Step Instructions:

1 **Prepare the base.**
   Put the cooked rice into 2 serving bowls.

2 **Make the tuna mix.**
   In a mixing bowl, add the drained tuna, coconut milk, pineapple (or mango), shredded carrot, and lime juice. Stir gently with a spoon. Add a pinch of salt.

3 **Assemble the bowl.**
   Spoon the tuna mixture on top of the rice in each bowl. Add a sprinkle of chopped cucumber or green onion if using.

4 **Serve and enjoy.**
   Eat with a spoon. Tastes great warm or chilled!

Tips for Accessibility:
Use a pull-top can of tuna or get help opening.
Use pre-cooked rice (microwave pouch) and pre-chopped fruit/veg.
All ingredients are soft—no chopping needed.

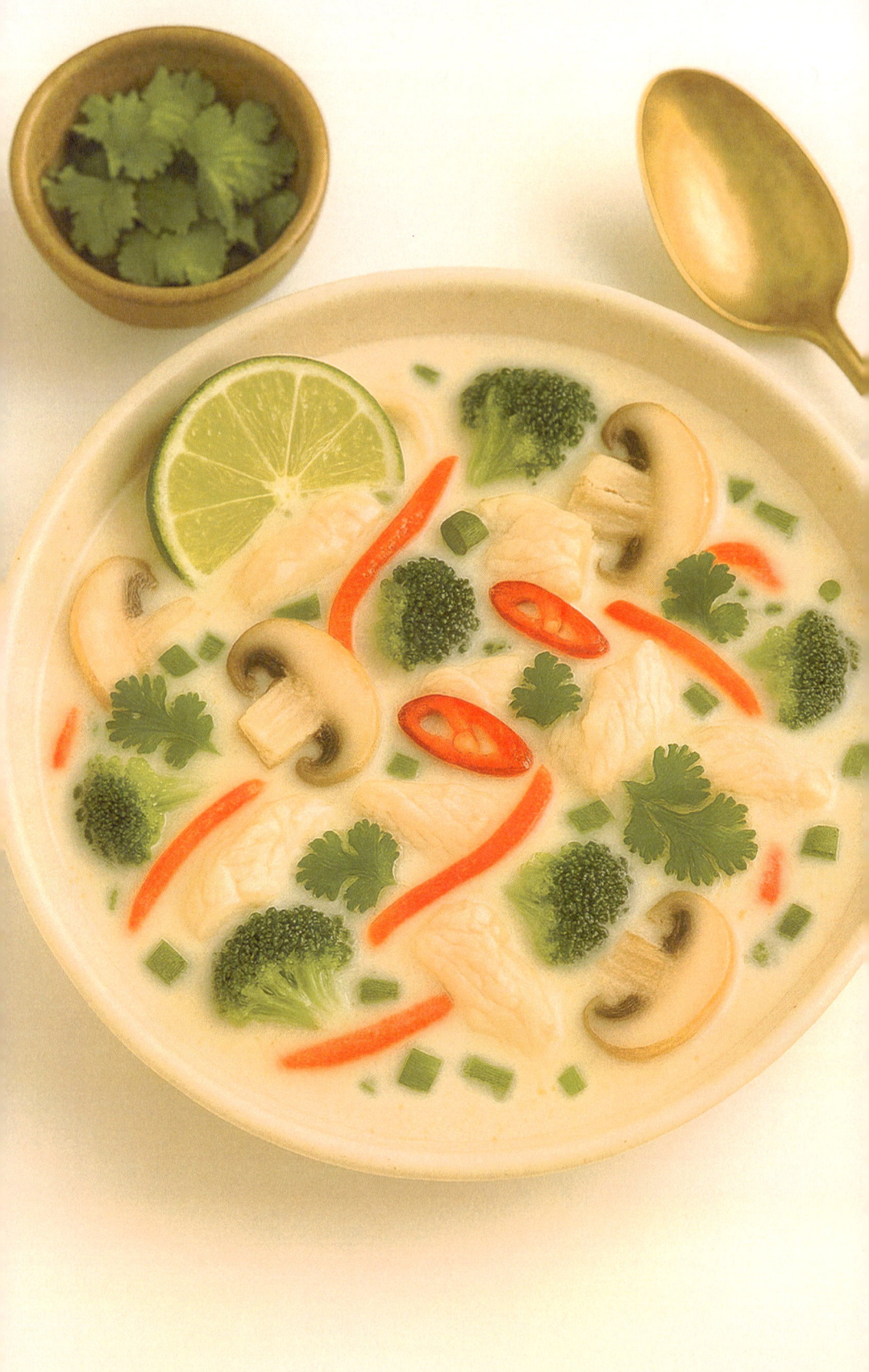

Thai Coconut Soup

The red curry, ginger, lemongrass, and coconut milk give this soup a delicious aroma and even more scrumptious taste. If you can't find shiitake mushrooms, button or cremini mushrooms will work in a pinch. You can find most of these ingredients in the Ethnic food aisle of your grocery store, but if you have a local Asian market to go to, even better.

Ingredients:

1 pound medium shrimp, peeled and deveined

4 cups chicken broth

3 13-ounce cans of coconut milk (regular or reduced fat)

½ pound fresh shiitake mushrooms (sliced)

1 tablespoon vegetable oil

2 tablespoons grated fresh ginger

1 stalk of lemongrass (minced)

2 teaspoons red curry paste

3 tablespoons fish sauce

1 tablespoon light brown sugar

¼ cup fresh cilantro (chopped)

Salt and pepper to taste

Tools You'll Need:

Large pot

Spoon

Measuring cups and spoons

Step-by-Step Instructions:

1 Start your soup.

Heat the oil in a large pot over medium heat. Stir in lemongrass, ginger, and curry paste for one minute until fragrant. Slowly pour the chicken broth over the mixture and stir continually. Stir in fish sauce and brown sugar, bring to a boil, then simmer for 15 minutes.

2 Finish your soup.

Stir in coconut milk and mushrooms, stirring until soft, about five minutes. Add in the shrimp and cook until no longer translucent, about five minutes. Stir in lemon juice and season with salt and pepper. Garnish with cilantro and serve immediately.

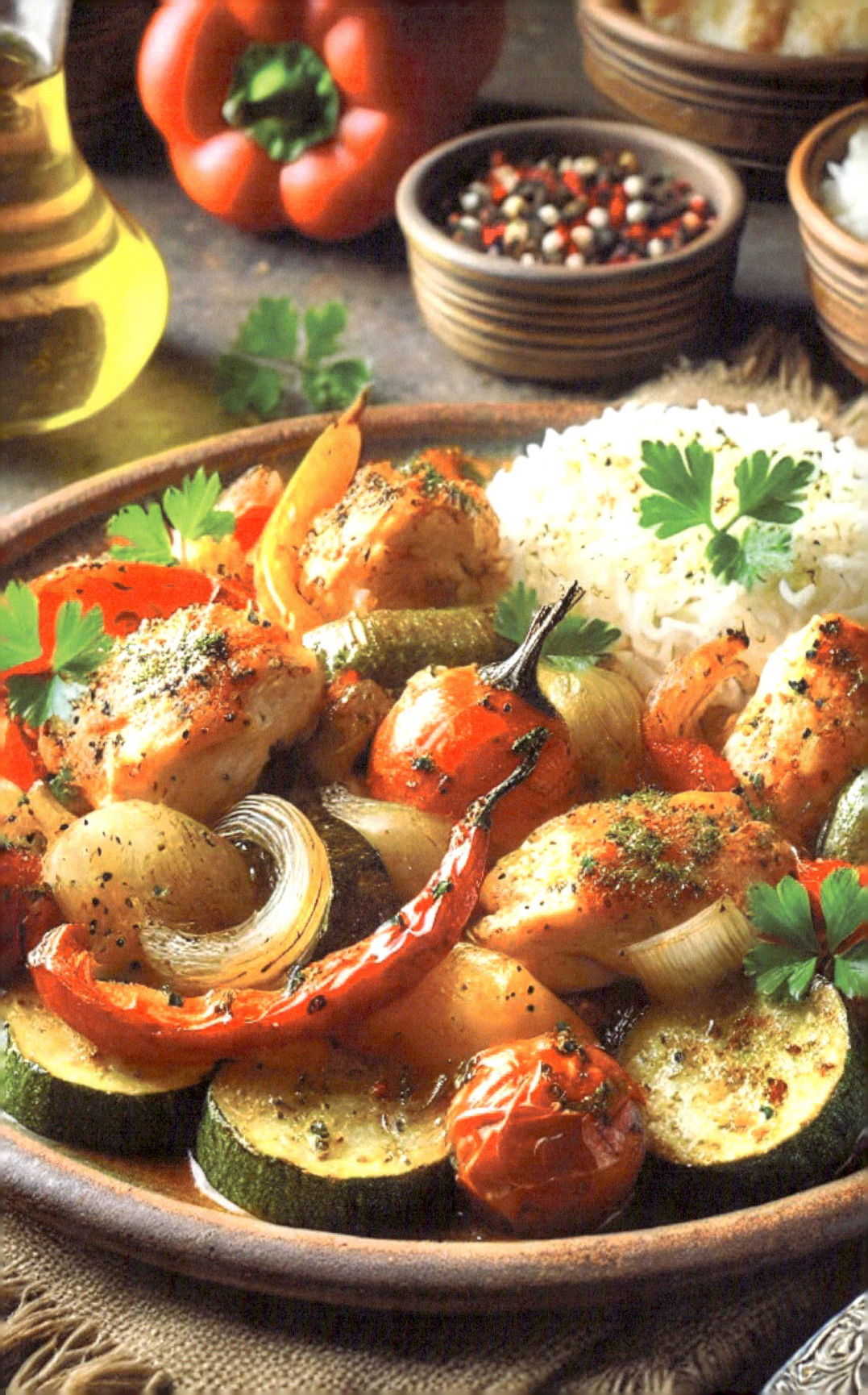

Turkish Chicken and Vegetables

This recipe features vibrant colors and juicy, flavorful chicken. I use bell peppers and potatoes, but you can substitute some other hearty vegetables like cauliflower or broccoli if that's what you have on hand. Serve with rice or salad.

Ingredients:
3 pounds of boneless, skinless chicken breasts
1 red bell pepper, sliced into strips
1 green bell pepper, sliced into strips
2 white onions (chopped)
6 Yukon Gold or Russet potatoes, peeled and chopped
1 can of diced tomatoes
½ cup of lemon juice
4 minced garlic cloves
1 ½ tablespoons of tomato paste
1 cup olive oil
1 tablespoon dried oregano
1 teaspoon salt
1 tablespoon black pepper

Tools You'll Need:
Large glass cooking dish
Paper towels
Measuring cups and spoons
Small bowl
Aluminum foil
Can opener

Tips for Accessibility:
Use pre-sliced chicken breast tenders and vegetables to avoid cutting.

Step-by-Step Instructions:

1 Preheat your oven to 375˚F and prepare the chicken.
Cut your chicken breasts into 8-10 pieces and dab with a paper towel. Season the chicken pieces with salt and pepper, then place them in a large, deep baking dish.

2 Add in vegetables and tomato paste.
Put in chopped onion, bell pepper, garlic, and chopped potatoes in the dish with the chicken, then pour the can of diced tomatoes on top. In a small bowl of hot water, dilute the tomato paste and add to the dish. Add the oregano, salt, and paper and give the contents of the dish a good stir.

3 Bake your chicken and vegetables.
Cover your tray with aluminum foil and bake in the oven for 90 minutes, then uncover the tray and cook for another 10-15 minutes to give your chicken a nice golden color. Serve alongside rice and/or salad.

INDEX

NOTES